Publisher
Marie Butler-Knight

Product Manager
Phil Kitchel

Managing Editor
Cari Luna

Acquisitions Editor
Mike Sanders

Book Producer
Lee Ann Chearney/Amaranth

Development Editor
Doris Cross

Senior Production Editor
Christy Wagner

Copy Editor
Fran Blauw

Cartoonist
Jody Schaeffer

Illustrator
Wendy Frost

Photographer
Saeid Lahouti

Photograph Model
Joan Budilovsky

Cover Designers
Mike Freeland
Kevin Spear

Book Designers
Scott Cook and Amy Adams of DesignLab

Indexer
Tonya Heard

Layout/Proofreading
Angela Calvert
Darin Crone
Svetlana Dominguez
Mary Hunt

Contents at a Glance

Contents

Foreword

The world-famous violinist Sir Yehudi Menuhin said about yoga that it is "a technique ideally suited to prevent physical and mental illness and to protect the body generally, developing an inevitable sense of self-reliance and assurance." Yoga did not make him a musical genius, but has given him energy, balance, and a sense of well-being for the past four decades, allowing him full expression of his great talent.

Yoga can do the same for anyone. Old or young. Male or female. Busy or super busy. In fact, yoga in one form or another is practiced by several million people today. It has been part of the kaleidoscope of our Western culture for over a century now and has proven incredibly effective in the maintenance of a sound body and mind and even the restoration of one's health. This is why several progressive insurance companies are now including yoga in their alternative therapies coverage.

Yoga is a tradition that looks back upon at least 5,000 years of experience and experimentation. Although it was created in India in a different cultural environment, the basic insights and laws on which it is based are valid anywhere in the world. Of course, there is much more to yoga than its potency as a system of health care. But this is for you to discover.

In this book, you will be gently but persuasively guided into the beginnings of yoga practice. The authors serve as knowledgeable and cheerful friends, motivating you all the way. Within these pages you will find no lack of encouragement, and everything is explained step by step. So, please, take the leap into what you will discover to be a rewarding and healing experience.

Georg Feuerstein, Ph.D., M. Litt.

Georg Feuerstein, Ph.D., M. Litt., is director of the Yoga Research Center; author of *Shambhala Encyclopedia of Yoga* and *Shambhala Guide to Yoga;* editor of the *Yoga World* newsletter; and a contributing editor of *Yoga Journal.*

Introduction

Imagine waking up one morning to find that all stresses in your life have been replaced with total joy. Yes, joy—the kind of pure joy you felt as a child when it was summer and the sun was shining and you had nothing to do but explore the whole world. Now, imagine possessing a strong, flexible body over which you have complete control. To top that off (literally!), imagine a mind free of chaotic thought, confusion, and uncertainty. Imagine pure health, pure consciousness, and pure bliss. These are the goals of the *yogi*.

And that *yogi* is you! Even if you don't attain your goals tomorrow or the next day, you will soon be on an amazing journey. We have each traveled down our own paths a little way. We've looked ahead, peeked over the horizon of the next few hills, and now we'd like to give you some hints about how to make the most of what's in store for you on your journey into yourself. Yoga is a process of self-discovery, and everyone's discoveries will be different, but we hope to steer you toward the potential "you," the perfect "you," the "you" waiting to be set free.

It won't be difficult. Yoga is beautifully simple. In fact, we think you're gonna love it!

How to Use This Book

This book is divided into seven parts, each bringing yoga into your life in a different way.

Part 1, "Let's Get Into Yoga," eases you into the concepts of yoga. We talk about why this ancient Eastern system of health is great for modern Westerners and how yoga can improve all aspects of your fitness, including your performance in other sports. We introduce you to your body, yoga-style, and reveal what yoga can do to improve your mental state as well as your physical condition.

Part 2, "Let's Get Spiritual: Growing with the Tree of Yoga," includes a little history, just to put yoga in context, then explains the various types of yoga. Next, we talk about the "rules" (yoga's guidelines for living), the importance of breath control, and the finer points of *Hatha Yoga*, the most popular form of yoga in the West.

Part 3, "Starting Your Yoga Practice," will help you do just that. We offer advice on how to find a yoga class and teacher, how to practice yoga at home, what to wear, how to overcome any mental stumbling blocks, when to practice, how to squeeze yoga into a busy day, and how to craft your own, personalized practice. This part of the book will help you make yoga your own.

Part 4, "Energize: Postures to Build Strength and Endurance," is the first part of exercises. We show you outstanding standing postures, beautiful backbends, terrific twists, and inversions, including the famous headstand posture. We'll also talk about *vinyasa*, dynamic combinations of postures that will have you breaking a sweat.

Part 5, "Calming Down: Postures to Quiet the Body and Mind," is the part of calming and centering postures, including sitting and meditative poses, forward bends, and a detailed discussion of *shavasana*, or the corpse pose. You'll learn how to let go of your mind, and you'll discover how great stress management can feel.

Part 6, "Living Your Yoga," is about specific aspects of the yoga lifestyle. We show you how to use *chakras*, *mudras*, *mantras*, and *mandalas* to enhance your yoga practice. We tell you the best foods for a *yogi* to eat and how yoga can address certain physical problems, from migraines to stomachaches and more.

Part 7, "Yoga for Everyone!" shows you how to practice yoga with a partner. You'll learn why yoga is great for all the stages in a woman's life, from PMS to menopause. We explain why yoga is a terrific practice for the whole family. Men will love and benefit from yoga, and you'll find out how to introduce yoga fun to your kids. Then, you'll discover how seniors can find renewed energy and health through yoga.

Yoga Jewels

Throughout this book, we've added four types of extra information in boxes, for your enlightenment:

Know Your Sanskrit

These boxes give you definitions for Sanskrit (the classical language of India) terms and correct pronunciations, too, so you can talk the talk.

A Yoga Minute

These boxes are full of fun anecdotes and trivia about the fascinating world of yoga.

Wise Yogi Tells Us

These special boxes offer you tips and advice for living your yoga.

Ouch!

These cautionary boxes contain information about how to avoid potential problems.

Acknowledgments

Far more people than can ever be mentioned here have, directly or indirectly, helped to make this book what it is. We'll name a few, but we send sincere and grateful energy out to all of you: Joan's dear friend and Webmaster Kathie Huddleston, who convinced her that she needed a yoga Web site on the Internet, and who consequently created the most beautiful YOYOGA! Web site (www.yoyoga.com). All Joan's students, who have taught and continue to teach her so much, and to all her many inspiring teachers along the way. Eve's children, Angus and Emmett, who are already accomplished *yogis* at the tender ages of five and two. Joan's foster children, who, however briefly they hold the key to her home, will forever hold the key to her heart. Joan's feline companions, Mufasa and Simba, who continually challenge vegetarian principles. Dr. Georg Feuerstein, for his invaluable advice and counsel. Saeid Lahouti, the photographer for this book, who has shared at least a few lifetimes with Joan (the photos for this book alone took several!). Wendy Frost, for her beautiful illustrations. Lee Ann Chearney at Amaranth, our book producer, for always giving us "all the best," and always promising "More soon!" Witty and charming Gary Krebs, for finding Joan on the Internet. The whole team at Alpha: Mike Sanders, Doris Cross, and Christy Wagner. William Hunt, for walking his talk, for being one of Joan's most inspiring teachers, and for his high-caliber tech review. Joan's friend, Bob Rumba, for hangin' in there through thick and thin, and in the deep and shallow waters of water yoga. Fr. Frank Stroud of Fordham University for increasing Joan's awareness in the awakened de Mello way. Eve's many supportive and appreciative *yogi* friends, including Jane deLaubenfels, Karen Woditsch, Kathy Streckfus, Caitlin Scott, Geo Takoma, the incomparable Katresha, and Jodi Komitor. Joan's friend, Chuck Reiter, whose simultaneous nostril breathing and continual encouragement are each appreciated in their own way. The many wonderful bookstores (the people in them, really) that have encouraged both of us as writers. Joan's parents, John and Leona, and Eve's parents, Richard and Penny. And to our families and friends who have been there or are there to lend an ear, a hand, a good thought, the right words, or whatever it takes—offering yet another view of the "many limbs" of yoga.

Special Thanks to the Technical Reviewer

The Complete Idiot's Guide to Yoga, Second Edition, was reviewed by an expert who checked the technical accuracy of what you'll learn here, to help us ensure that this book gives you everything you need to know about yoga. Special thanks are extended to William Hunt.

William Hunt is a certified yoga instructor, ordained priest, and the director of the *Hatha Yoga* teacher's training program at the Temple of Kriya Yoga in Chicago. He also co-teaches with Dr. Bruno Cortis, cardiologist, in wellness seminars.

Special Thanks to the Book Producer

This book would not have been possible without the expert vision and editorial guidance of Lee Ann Chearney of Amaranth. The team at Alpha is immeasurably grateful to her for her hard work and diligence. Thanks, Lee Ann!

Trademarks

All terms mentioned in this book that are known to be or are suspected of being trademarks or service marks have been appropriately capitalized. Alpha Books and Macmillan USA, Inc., cannot attest to the accuracy of this information. Use of a term in this book should not be regarded as affecting the validity of any trademark or service mark.

Part 1
Let's Get Into Yoga

Part 1 is an introduction and more, filling you in on why the ancient and venerable system of living called yoga is so relevant to our modern Western world. If you want to get in better physical, mental, emotional, and spiritual shape, yoga is the key. No matter what your fitness level, no matter what your personal philosophy, no matter what your religion or lack thereof, yoga can make a positive impact on your life.

We go on to help you get more familiar with your body, and on better terms with the body you call your own. We also show you what yoga can do for your body's strength, flexibility, balance, grace, and muscle tone. Do you know whether you are an ectomorph, an endomorph, or a mesomorph, and what each of those terms means? You will after reading Chapter 3, "How Comfortable Are You in Your Body?" Chapter 4, "Yoga Mind Power: Go with the Flow," ends this part with a little mind power. Learn how yoga can make your mind as toned, strong, sharp, and effective as it makes your body strong and supple. Learn what yoga's true and original purpose has always been, and how this ultimate objective can lift you to a new level of personal achievement. Best of all, learn how yoga can set you free to feel and enjoy pure, unfettered bliss.

Chapter 1

Why Practice Yoga?

In This Chapter

➤ Learn what yoga is

➤ How yoga helps alleviate stress

➤ Using yoga to promote strength, balance, and flexibility

➤ Using yoga as preventive medicine

When it comes to yoga, idiots just don't exist. Banish the thought that yoga is too esoteric to understand, too mystical, or on the fringe. Forget about the notion that yoga is only for double-jointed people who've been able to fold themselves into a suitcase since birth, or for perpetual 1960s flower children who sit around and chant all day. Negative thinking and stereotypes are contrary to the philosophy of yoga; yoga is user friendly. Anyone—at any fitness level, and with a wide range of personal and fitness goals—can benefit from beginning a yoga practice. Even you.

Maybe you want to try yoga because you've never been able to touch your toes and you'd like to do it before you retire. Maybe you're seeking a quiet place to center yourself, to meditate by taking your mind somewhere far away from the house, the kids, the office, and the million nagging details of everyday life. Maybe you're an athlete who wants to learn yoga breathing for the advantage gained by stronger lungs and better circulation. Or maybe you've heard that yoga is great for migraine headaches, relief from chronic lower back pain, or good physical therapy after an injury or during an illness. It's all true.

The ancient and venerable art of yoga is neither a sport nor a religion; it's a journey of the body and mind. When you do yoga, you nurture the movement of *prana*—the life force. You'll read a lot of Sanskrit words in this book because yoga terminology originated thousands of years ago in this ancient language. But there's nothing ancient about the concept of *prana*: *Prana* is the life "force." May the force be with you as you begin your yoga practice.

What Is Yoga?

Yoga is a system of techniques that reflects real and proven scientific concepts. Many things Western scientists understand about the body have actually been known by yoga practitioners for centuries. Yoga sees the body from a different perspective than traditional Western medicine, but the basic principles are the same. What we Westerners call *nerve plexus*, yoga calls *chakras* (although these terms don't coincide precisely—*chakras* include psychospiritual energy). What we Westerners call *spinal alignment*, yoga accomplishes through various poses or exercises designed to do what many of us pay chiropractors to do. The human body is in a constant state of flux, continually adjusting internally to the influence of a changing external environment. Western medicine calls this process *homeostasis*. Yoga's *five sheaths of existence*—in essence, the body, the breath, the emotions, the intellect, and happiness—reflect the same need for balance between internal and external forces. The terminology may be different, but the concepts are universal.

Know Your Sanskrit

Yoga (pronounced *YOH-gah*) is derived from the Sanskrit root *yuj,* meaning "to yoke or join together." **Prana** (*PRAH-nah*) is a form of energy in the universe that animates all physical matter, including the human body. *Prana* is the soul of the universe. Doing yoga maximizes your body's flow of the universal life force, giving you better health and increased vitality. **Chakras** (*CHAH-krahs*) are centers of energy located between the base of your spinal column and the crown of your head. Each *chakra* has a corresponding color, sound, perception, and biological function. Note that the actual spelling of *chakra* is *cakra,* but this spelling isn't commonly used.

Yoga is a fun activity that can produce powerful results. Yoga will wake up your body, sharpen your mind, and clarify your spirit. Yoga doesn't hurt, is only as difficult as you make it, and allows you to proceed at an individualized pace. Yoga can be a tiny part of your life; or you can incorporate its theories, rituals, postures, diet, and philosophy into every aspect of your life. You control how deeply yoga touches you. But if you begin a steady practice, be assured that yoga will transform the way you look, feel, move, breathe, and interact with friends, family, and co-workers.

Yoga Is Occident Insurance

Life in the West (the Occident, as opposed to the Orient) is no picnic. Sure, it's exciting, even exhilarating, but after all the pressures, stresses, responsibilities, frustrations, resentments, choices, temptations, and obsessions the average Westerner has faced by the end of a typical working day, it's no wonder we are a culture eagerly searching for ways to simplify our lives.

So how can yoga help? In the face of a daily existence that is so vibrant it almost vibrates us apart, yoga is an oasis. Yoga teaches the frantic mind to settle and find peace, and it helps the ravaged body to heal itself by optimizing our natural ability to heal, and by building physical confidence as well as emotional well-being. Yoga removes scattered energy, replaces depleted energy, and keeps your body, including all its internal systems, toned and in good working order.

Ouch!

Yoga doesn't hurt and isn't about unnatural contortion. Sure, accomplished *yogis* may be able to move into seemingly impossible positions, but these postures are for people who have progressed to a level where such positions are possible and helpful. Some bodies are born more flexible than others. Each person has to find his or her own edge—the point just before discomfort occurs—and grow into it at a comfortable pace. We're all working the same edge, just in different places!

So … what are we getting at here, you ask? Yoga is the best life insurance policy there is. It helps you slow down, center yourself, and get the most out of your life so that every day is precious. By holding the body in a series of yoga postures that stretch and strengthen your muscles, loosen your joints, focus your breathing, and tone your internal organs, you'll find a new friend in your body. While you continue to hold each posture, your mind will learn how to tune out the distractions of life and hone in on how things are for you in this moment of living. Doing yoga makes you *listen* to how you feel—physically and mentally. This newfound power of concentration will carry over into every aspect of your life. Signals you once ignored—that crick in your neck or your obsessive worrying over a detail that keeps you from seeing the forest for the trees—are instantly acknowledged and seen for what they are: warning signs that you are heading down the wrong path. Yoga can help you regain your sense of self-fulfillment and joy, ensuring a more satisfying, not to mention fitter, existence.

Yoga Is a Great Stress Buster

Stress is a simple fact of life on earth in the twenty-first century; stress is so common that countries all over the globe are incorporating the English word "stress" into their own languages: "*Que* stress. ¡Me siento agobiada/o!" (translation from Spanish: "*What* stress. I am totally overwhelmed!"). If you've never been under stress, we'd like to know your secret. (It's probably yoga!)

Know Your Sanskrit

Asanas (pronounced *AH-sah-nahs*) are the postures, or exercises, of yoga designed to help you master control of your body. Asanas are also meant to facilitate meditation. *Pranayama* (*PRAH-nah-YAH-mah*) are breathing exercises designed to help you master control of your breath.

Yoga tackles stress on many levels. The postures, or *asanas,* help you control your wayward body, making it stronger, more flexible, better functioning, and consequently, more resistant to disease and other physical problems. Practicing the *asanas* trains your body to do exactly what you tell it to do. Your doctor knows that moderate exercise, deep breathing, and relaxation are all great ways to relieve stress—yoga accomplishes all three. Yoga's breathing exercises, or *pranayama,* consciously channel the flow of the life force, *prana,* into and out of the body. Physiologically, deep, regular breathing sends a signal to each cell of your body to relax. Yoga meditation calms your racing thoughts and exercises your ability to master your own mind, rather than let your mind master you.

Yoga is a physical, mental, and spiritual way of life that puts reality into perspective. Yoga doesn't change your stressful circumstances, but it does teach you how to react to them without neglecting or injuring yourself.

Yoga Promotes Whole-Body Fitness

Maybe you're an accomplished athlete, or maybe you're a couch potato. Exercise to you may mean breezing through a five-mile run in the morning and a requisite visit to the gym three times a week, or it may mean getting up to look for the remote control. Either way, yoga is perfect for you!

Because yoga combines so many different fitness elements and is so easily tailored to the individual, it can be practiced with great benefit at the beginner level as well as at the most advanced level. Whether you're a beginning or advanced practitioner, yoga will slowly, gently, and easily open up your body. You'll feel taller, breathe easier, and move about more comfortably.

Nonathletes also might be attracted to the idea that yoga isn't competitive. In fact, a sense of competitiveness is in direct opposition to the yoga frame of mind. Your yoga practice is personal and has nothing to do with anybody else. Plus, yoga will give you so much energy and such an improved self-image that you may find exercise isn't as bad as you thought.

Yoga is designed to work all your muscles, not just a few isolated major muscle groups. Many of the postures, such as the twists and inversions, stimulate particular internal organs or release energy from stress-prone areas such as the lower back or neck. Yoga's fine-tuning exercises are the ultimate full-body workout. Other exercise programs tend to develop only one part of you—cardiovascular fitness, leg strength, or fat burning, for example. Yoga does it all.

Although many types of yoga exist, *Hatha Yoga* is the branch of yoga that concentrates on the body and is the form of yoga most emphasized in this book and practiced by Westerners. *Hatha Yoga* is an excellent fitness program, but it's also more. *Hatha Yoga* is based on the idea that gaining supreme control over your body is the key to control of your mind and freedom of your spirit. Through postures (*asanas*), breathing exercises (*pranayama*), and meditation, *Hatha Yoga* exercises, tones, and strengthens the whole person—body, mind, and spirit. Even if you start with the physical exercises alone, however, *Hatha Yoga* will quickly begin to work its magic.

A Yoga Minute

According to the National Heart, Lung, and Blood Institute, heart disease is almost twice as likely to develop in physically inactive people.

Know Your Sanskrit

Hatha Yoga (pronounced *HAT-ha YOH-gah*, not *HATH-ah YOH-gah*, as it is frequently mispronounced) is the type of yoga most commonly practiced in Western culture. *Ha* means "sun," and *tha* means "moon," so *hatha* is a combining of complementary forces. *Hatha Yoga* is the branch of yoga that transforms the human body via physical strengthening and purification to make the body a worthy vehicle of self-realization.

Fitness today means more than a healthy body. Our culture is experiencing a growing trend toward things spiritual. With a growing passion for holistic health alternatives, we are a society looking for balance in a world that is out of balance. Holistic fitness is quickly becoming a mainstream concept, and yoga fits comfortably into this trend. Yoga is the answer to the spiritual seeker's *and* the athlete's search for physical excellence, because it's the best all-purpose, all-person, whole-self, individualized fitness program—time-tested over centuries.

Yoga Is Healing Power

Yoga is a boon to the healthy body, but it can also be of supreme benefit to the body in need of healing. Of course, the best route for a healthy person to take is one of prevention. Healthy habits, maintenance of the body, peacefulness of mind, and calmness of spirit will go a long way toward protecting you from compromised health. Yoga is great preventive medicine, because it keeps all of you—body, mind, attitude, outlook, immune system—in top form. Your spine, the "Grand Central Station" of your body, is stretched, loosened, and aligned by yoga—postures are designed to allow energy to flow freely through your spine and entire body. Many holistic health practitioners and even traditional practitioners argue that if the spine is aligned, the entire body works better, feels better, and fights disease more effectively.

Yoga aids …

➤ Circulation.

➤ Digestion.

➤ Respiration.

➤ Reproduction.

Yoga also …

➤ Tones your organs.

➤ Improves your posture.

➤ Frees your breathing.

➤ Is cleansing.

Yoga helps your body purge itself of toxins that can negatively affect your health, both by releasing negative energy and, more directly, removing obstacles to the proper stimulation of the body's *lymphatic system*. The lymphatic system, the centerpiece of the immune system, protects and maintains the body's internal fluid environment, both filtering toxins and transporting nutrients to the blood. Lymph is pumped through the body by movement—when we breathe, contract or release our muscles, or even with the motion of our beating hearts or our digestive systems as we process food we've eaten. Yoga helps our bodies go with their natural flow. Even if you're not very mobile, you can practice yoga with eye exercises, simple stretches, and conscious rhythmic movements. Take your fitness personally and craft a yoga fitness plan that is all your own.

If you're sick, injured, or bothered by nagging health complaints, yoga can be a therapeutic addition to your physician's treatment plan. Of course, yoga should *never* be used in place of competent medical care. Ask your doctor or physical therapist about how yoga can be helpful in alleviating your specific health problems or concerns.

A Yoga Minute

According to the World Health Organization, an estimated 691 million people worldwide suffer from high blood pressure.

My Yogi, Myself

Once you've created your yoga plan and have begun to practice, guess what you are? Healthier? Sure. In better shape? Of course. But you're something else, too—you're a *yogi!* (A female *yogi* is actually called a *yogini*, pronounced *YOH-gee-nee*, but let's be contemporary and say we're all *yogis*.) Anyone who practices yoga is a *yogi*—that's what *yogi* means. You needn't be wise, you don't have to wear a loincloth, and you certainly don't need to practice for 10 hours every day. Even if you start with just a little yoga, you're a *yogi*. Of course, the more yoga you practice, the more you'll gain, and the wiser a *yogi* you'll become.

Yoga is practiced to varying degrees around the world, but some exuberant practitioners who have devoted their lives to the practice of yoga have achieved amazing control over their bodies. Although, according to yoga, such feats aren't important to the goal of spiritual enlightenment (self-realization), *yogis* have been known to …

➤ Stop their own hearts (then start them again, of course).

➤ Live to be well over 100 years old.

➤ Suspend their breath for an hour a day or more.

➤ Stand on one foot for several years (don't ask us why).

➤ Lie comfortably on a bed of nails.

➤ Eat razor blades without harm (we prefer a nice salad).

Here are a few more incredible feats that border on the supernatural, but these we'd have to see to believe:

➤ Become invisible at will.

➤ Remain suspended in mid-air (handy when all the chairs are taken).

➤ Move through space at the speed of light (saves on gasoline).

It doesn't matter why you approach yoga—whether for fitness, stress relief, enlightenment, or healing. It doesn't matter how advanced you are, whether you are out of shape and inflexible or an athlete extraordinaire. It certainly doesn't matter how much you already know about yoga. If you let yoga help you, it will help you in whatever way you require.

If you're intrigued but still need just a little more convincing before you're ready to perform pretzel-like contortions or begin *dhyana* (your daily meditation), read on for 10 great reasons to practice yoga:

Know Your Sanskrit

Dhyana (pronounced *dee-YAH-nah*) means "meditation"—the process of quieting the mind to free yourself from preconceptions and illusions. The result is a clearer vision of the truth about yourself, your life, and the world. For more on meditation in its many forms, read *The Complete Idiot's Guide to Meditation,* by the authors of this book.

➤ Yoga will tone your muscles and trim excess weight. It may even change your attitude about your body for the better.

➤ Anyone can do yoga. It's just a matter of starting at the appropriate level and remembering that you aren't competing with anyone.

➤ Yoga doesn't hurt. You go at your own pace, do what feels good, and stop before you feel pain. What could be better?

➤ Yoga will give you the gift of boundless energy.

➤ The increased energy and vitality you receive from regular yoga practice will make you feel as if hours have been added to your day.

➤ Yoga lets you dare to be different. People who tease you about doing yoga don't understand what you're doing—explain it to them!

➤ You can do as much or as little yoga as you like. Start with the postures, and you may find that your interest in breathing, chanting, and meditation develops later—or not at all, which is fine, too. It's all up to you.

➤ Yoga is definitely not about guilt! You can benefit the most from regular yoga practice, but practicing the postures whenever you have time is still beneficial and certainly better than no yoga at all.

➤ Contrary to popular belief, yoga isn't a religion. It's a method for life that can complement and enhance any religious system of beliefs, or it can be practiced completely apart from religion.

➤ Yoga will help ease your aches, pains, and stiffness. You'll feel like a kid again.

But don't take being a *yogi* lightly just because you've become one without too much effort. Your body, your mind, and your happiness are *your* responsibility. Your yoga program is a great start, but you need to have the right yoga plan. Learn as much as you can about yoga, and consider taking a yoga class. The best way to learn yoga is with a teacher who can help you with the finer points of the postures, answer your individual questions, and guide you in finding a sequence of postures that best suit your needs and personality.

Even before you find a teacher, though, reading and learning about yoga can start you on your way. The more you know about yoga, the more you can focus on how it can help you. This book is a great start in your search for the perfectly personalized program. Apply everything you learn to your own journey. How can each new piece of information improve the personal program you are creating for yourself? Think about what you've learned already. Are you beginning to see how yoga might fit into your life? Yes? Then you are wiser already.

Wise Yogi Tells Us

If you are overweight or have a problem with overeating, yoga is the perfect exercise for you; it's gentle on the out-of-shape body, stiff joints, and heart. You'll feel better about your body as you begin to lose weight, and you can achieve an inner peace and confidence that will help you avoid compulsive overeating.

Yoga Sets You Free

Perhaps you're flirting with the idea of yoga because you imagine it's an interesting fitness plan, but perhaps you're looking for something more. People have been practicing yoga for thousands of years, not because they want to be "in shape" (a fringe benefit), but because they are seeking meaning in life. Yoga can be a fitness program, but it can also be a path to greater self-knowledge and, ultimately, self-actualization. Yoga helps you reach the fullness of your human potential. You will be more confident, stronger, healthier, and more at peace with who you are. You will make better decisions, set and achieve worthwhile goals, and become the person you want to be.

The ultimate goal of the *yogi* is to achieve the experience of truth, which may mean different things to different people, but which is, to some degree, a consistent experience for all—a clarity of vision, supreme focus, and a feeling of oneness with the earth, even the universe. This ideal state

Know Your Sanskrit

Samadhi (pronounced *sah-MAH-dee*) is the goal of yoga. It's when the *yogi* finally becomes aware of nothing but *brahman* (*BRAH-mahn*)—the all-pervading Supreme Self, or God—everywhere. It's a state of absolute bliss and may be transitory or, ideally, perpetual.

is called *samadhi* and involves consciousness to such a heightened degree that individual ego falls away, and oneness with the universal force of love and goodness, or *brahman,* is achieved. It is the state of pure bliss.

A few rare and diligent *yogis* have been able to maintain this state for extended periods, but for most of us, *samadhi* is an elusive experience. We may get occasional glimpses of it, or sudden rushes of bliss that fall away but become imprinted in our memories. After all, we do have to live in the world, which is often a less-than-blissful place. On the other hand, you and your world are what you make them, and yoga can help you optimize yourself, your experience, and your all-important perception of the world around you. Yoga is fitness plus peace and fitness plus joy.

The Least You Need to Know

➤ Yoga reduces stress and improves concentration.

➤ Yoga is a great workout at any fitness level.

➤ Yoga helps prevent illness and keeps the systems of the body in order.

➤ Yoga increases energy and vitality, promoting well-being.

➤ Anyone who practices yoga is a *yogi!*

Chapter 2

Yoga Fitness Power: Beyond Stretching

In This Chapter

➤ Yoga as a body/mind workout

➤ Yoga as your ultimate fitness power source

➤ Cross-train with yoga

➤ How yoga enhances your sports performance

Yoga is more than stretching. No matter what your fitness level, yoga can be a challenging exercise program that builds superior strength and endurance. You'll even break a sweat! Yoga involves a level of mental and physical concentration that results in greater flexibility, increased muscle power, refined balance, improved cardiovascular function, increased lung capacity, toned immune and digestive systems, and improved functioning of internal organs. If you're looking to yoga for body/mind fitness power, you've come to the right place.

Yoga Means Connection

Yoga taps into your inner power, connecting your body with your mind. It's easy to fall into a pattern of associating fitness with the body alone. We run, do aerobic dance, bicycle, and perform sit-ups and pushups—all for our bodies. What does your mind have to do with it? But the *yogi* will soon see the absurdity of this notion. Body and mind are one, and although they can become isolated and dissociated from each other, yoga brings them back together where they belong. Everything works better when all the circuits are connected. Your mind can boost your physical performance to new heights, and control over your body is training for control over your mind.

Are You Off Balance?

Perhaps you've been feeling "scattered" lately. Do you lose things easily? Forget appointments or information? Are you overwhelmed by the buzz of activity in your life? Maybe you think you don't have the time to slow down and get "centered," but you must know this: You don't have the time *not* to get centered. If you're feeling out of balance, you're wasting your days, your energy, and your power. You're like a house with the heat on and all the windows open. Yoga can help you close the windows (or turn off the heat) and center on making the most of each precious moment of your day.

Sometimes stress is a good thing. It can give you the power to escape from a dangerous situation. It can help you succeed in life, both in your physical pursuits (say, running a marathon) and in your intellectual challenges (say, passing a test). Too much stress, however, wreaks havoc on the body. When experiencing stress, the brain stimulates the adrenal glands, resulting in certain telltale symptoms:

➤ Your heart rate speeds up.

➤ Your blood pressure rises.

➤ Your breathing quickens and becomes more shallow.

➤ Your pupils dilate.

➤ Your muscles tense.

➤ You sweat.

➤ Your senses become heightened.

➤ Blood flows to your muscles and brain.

Too much of this kind of activity will wear out anyone's system. Yoga's body/mind fitness power can channel stress more efficiently, helping you instead of hurting you.

Mind Meet Body, Body Meet Mind

Beginning to practice yoga is like introducing your body and your mind for the first time. Sure, they have resided in close proximity your entire life, but do they really know each other? If you want to be truly fit, you must introduce your body to your mind and your mind to your body. *Hatha Yoga*, the yoga that concentrates on strengthening and purifying the physical body, is the perfect introduction.

Practicing *Hatha Yoga* means finding the balance in the union of your body, mind, and spirit. *Hatha Yoga* is truly a holistic exercise (body + mind + spirit = holistic), because it involves the activation, control, and mastery of every part of your body. Fitness is the inevitable result—so is restful sleep, improved health, and tranquillity of mind. *Hatha Yoga* gives voice to what the body knows: All its parts are one.

Coming Back to Center

Just like any other sport, yoga requires a warm-up period. Haphazardly practicing may build your strength to a small degree, but you won't get the benefits of yoga's body/mind discipline. Centering is a mental warm-up to go along with your physical warm-up. As you practice your beginning poses, consciously focus your mind on your body. Notice how your body feels and what it's doing. Commit to your yoga practice for the next 10, 15, 30, or however many minutes you have allotted yourself. The more often you make a habit of consciously centering your mind on what your body is doing, the more you'll notice a feeling of calm, of being centered in your daily life. Your yoga fitness power is showing!

Ouch!

If you have a medical condition, such as chronic back pain, yoga can be great therapy. A yoga teacher can show you which postures will benefit and strengthen your particular weak area. But be careful: The postures should feel comfortable, not painful!

Tapping Into Your Yoga Power Source

So how does all this "centering" and concentration get you in shape? Because your mind and your body are so intricately connected, a centered mind with the power of concentration works directly on the body, allowing each yoga posture to accomplish the maximum possible benefit. Don't be misled into thinking you can ignore the "mental" parts of yoga because you aren't in it for the "enlightenment." Perhaps getting in shape is priority one for you. That's great! But the key to yoga's fitness power is in the synthesis of everything you are: your body, your mind, your spirit—each part working together to make the whole stronger, healthier, and more alive. Remember, a healthy body means more than just a strong body. As any doctor will tell you, a positive attitude toward life is central to the body's natural healing powers. Yoga stimulates your body/mind power source, channeling your positive mental energy into your physical workout, and vice versa.

Bend Without Breaking

If you've always been athletic but haven't concentrated on maintaining your flexibility, you may be nervous about trying yoga. You may ask yourself, "Don't I have to be able to sit in that *lotus pose* all day?" Of course not! Endurance isn't necessary for the beginning runner—you attain endurance by running. Yoga is the same way. If you're about as flexible as a steel pole, start slowly and go only as far into a posture as you can. Every week of practice will take you farther. Before you know it, your joints will loosen, your muscles will stretch, and your body will take on a smoother, more pleasing shape.

Know Your Sanskrit

The **lotus pose,** also called **_padmasana_** (pronounced *PAHD-MAH-sahn-ah*) is a yoga sitting pose in which the left foot lies upturned on the right thigh, and the right foot lies up-turned on the left thigh. It is meant to resemble the perfect symmetry and beauty of the lotus flower.

Perhaps you've always been naturally flexible. Don't think yoga will be simple! There's always the next posture waiting for you.

As you accomplish postures you couldn't begin to achieve when you started, you'll understand flexibility in a new way. The achievement of a yoga posture is like winning a marathon without anyone else losing—pure triumph!

Balancing Acts

You probably take your ability to balance for granted. You get up in the morning, walk around all day without incident, and lie back down at night. Balancing wasn't always so easy, however. In fact, during one illustrious period of your life, learning to balance took up most of your waking moments.

Through yoga, balancing once again captures your attention. Balance is challenging. Yoga balance postures take keen muscle control and strength, mental centering, and lots of practice. Once you've refined your balancing act, you'll discover that the walking you take for granted is even easier than before. Balancing is control, both in stillness and in motion.

Strength from the Gut

Everybody knows that lifting a heavy weight takes strength. But balancing takes strength, too. So does holding a posture for an extended time. Yoga strength training is *isometric* (a form of exercise in which muscles are tensed in opposition to each other or to an immovable object). After assuming each yoga pose, you hold it for as long as you can hold it correctly. Talk about a way to wake up muscles you never knew you had! Yoga's isometric action is easier on your muscles than the weight-bearing and pounding of other sports, yet extremely effective for building strength. What's more, each yoga position in a well-structured workout includes a posture and its opposite, so your body will stay physically centered, never developing any side or particular body part out of proportion to the others.

Yoga positions are entered and held by the body in order to find the peace within—the point where sustaining the pose is easy, natural, and feels "right." The more difficult the pose, the harder it is to find peace. Yoga postures mirror life. When things are easy, it's easy to feel good. But feeling good when things aren't going your way—whether it's a bad hair day or a serious tragedy—is a challenge. Yoga is a journey through the poses, working with each pose until you find that peace, then progressing to the next level. This progression combines the building of physical strength with the toning of the mind.

This might surprise the Western athlete even more: Strength is compounded when the body, mind, and spirit are exercised together. Strength will mean more to you, once you've practiced yoga, than it did before.

Keeping the Faith

"But I know it will be just like that aerobics class," you may be thinking. "I'll be all excited for the first week or two, then I'll get bored and quit." In any given day, probably just as many people quit a fitness program as start one. Why should yoga be any different?

The benefits you'll soon feel from your yoga practice are so comprehensive, you may well find that you'd rather give up coffee, doughnuts, or pepperoni pizza than give up your daily yoga "therapy." Beyond the more obvious benefits of increased flexibility, balance, and strength, yoga has thousands of less dramatic (though no less important) rewards. Yoga feels different than other fitness programs, because each posture is specifically designed to activate your body in minute ways—adjusting here, stimulating there, stretching here, strengthening there, compressing, releasing, expanding, and reaching. With all this internal maintenance, you can't help but enjoy increased health and a vibrant sense of well-being.

Yoga vs. Other Exercise

Most Western forms of exercise emphasize stress on the muscles combined with quick, harsh movements. Yoga avoids such movements, which tend to trigger lactic acid production in muscle fibers, leading to pain. In addition, yoga's emphasis on breathing delivers more oxygen to muscles to further lessen the effects of lactic acid production. You needn't give up your favorite sport, however.

Wise Yogi Tells Us

Yoga is great for teenagers, who already tend to be strong, flexible, and energetic. Teenagers are frequently surprised at how challenging yoga can be. The mental focus, physical control, and spiritual development that come along with yoga are wonderful therapies for adolescents whose hormones are raging and who may feel depressed, out of control, or angry, without knowing why.

Just add yoga to the program. But first, read on to see how yoga compares to your favorite fitness activity.

Yoga can enhance your performance in all your favorite sports.

Awesome Aerobics

Aerobic dance can be a lot of fun, especially for those who like music. Aerobic dancers who also do yoga are more graceful, have more fluid movements, are better able to keep up, and are more flexible. Like running, aerobic dance is primarily a cardiovascular activity; although low-impact aerobics are kinder to your body than high-impact, aerobic dancers still experience a lot of stress on their muscles and joints. Aerobics is energizing and great for people who need the motivation of a class and an instructor (something a yoga class also offers). Yoga is a great complement, because it balances aerobic dance's frenetic energy by inducing a sense of calm and inner control.

Rockin' Running

"But I *know* yoga won't give me the cardiovascular strength and endurance that running gives me!" you may be protesting. Consider this: Runners rely on strength and balance. Flexible runners get injured less often. Runners also tend to have shallow, hard breathing patterns; they sometimes hyperventilate. Yoga's deep breathing exercises increase your lung capacity, getting more oxygen to your brain and increasing your endurance.

Yoga is kinder to your body than running, so it makes a great alternate workout to give your body a rest from the constant pounding and joint stress runners experience. Runners frequently injure their feet, ankles, knees, and hips. You can use yoga postures to build strength in these same body parts! In fact, the New York Road Runners club promotes an official yoga program called "Power Yoga."

Super-Charged Stretching

Most of us have had basic stretching exercises drilled into us since grade school gym class. Bend down and touch your toes, reach to the right, reach to the left, roll your head from front to side to side. The difference between this type of stretching and yoga is that yoga stretches are specifically designed not only to lengthen your muscles, but also to stabilize your joints, stimulate your organs, balance your endocrine system, and strengthen your muscles as you hold the stretch. It's still a good idea to do basic stretches before engaging in strenuous exercise, such as running or swimming, but if you also add yoga to your fitness program, stretching will soon be a breeze.

A Yoga Minute

According to the National Sporting Goods Association, exercise walking was the number-one fitness activity in 1999, with 80.8 million participants. The sport that grew in popularity the most? Kickboxing, by a landslide.

Superior Swimming

Swimming is an excellent exercise, because it works your muscles and your heart without putting stress on your body. Swimming is essentially a cardiovascular exercise. You move through the water and increase your heart rate. If you're a swimmer, you'll find yoga a great addition to your fitness program, because the increased flexibility and strength gained through yoga make swimming easier. Also, the breathing practice in yoga is of exceptional benefit to swimmers, who must have good control over their breathing.

Uplifting Weight Lifting

Lifting weights adds bulk to muscles but decreases flexibility. Many weight-lifters are "muscle-bound." Weight-lifters can benefit dramatically from yoga: While weight training builds bone, muscle mass, and strength, yoga lengthens the muscles and keeps them flexible. Weight-lifters also benefit from the breathing exercises and balance training of yoga. Yoga is really a form of weight lifting. You aren't lifting barbells, but in many of the poses, you are lifting your own weight. Think about how much you weigh—wouldn't it be quite an accomplishment to lift that weight easily?

Wise Yogi Tells Us

End every yoga session with a few minutes of complete and total relaxation. Don't move, don't think; practice sitting or lying absolutely still. Simply feel your body. This little space at the end of your yoga workout is an important part of bringing mind and body together—grounding your awareness and allowing your body to make the most of your workout.

Ecstasy: Yoga Union

The Western approach to yoga tends to be more fitness-oriented, while the Eastern approach to yoga is based on the idea that a healthy body makes it easier to progress spiritually. Either approach benefits both body and mind, however. If you're interested in yoga for its physical benefits, you can consider the spiritual "centeredness" you achieve a splendid bonus. Or, if you tend more toward the Eastern way, consider fitness the icing on the cake of spiritual growth. Either way, yoga fitness power means self-confidence, self-control, and inner peace. Whatever your fitness level, let yoga challenge you.

It's All in Your Mind!

Everyone knows that a good percentage of athletic performance is mental. We've all seen our favorite team in a pressure situation get psyched out—suddenly, it can't do anything right. Think about the last time you played your favorite sport. Was there ever a time when you suddenly slipped into "the zone"? Your performance becomes flawless, and you're able to exceed your normal abilities.

Because yoga unites body and mind, it teaches you control over your mental state as it teaches you control over your body. What happens to you really is "all in your mind," so let your mind be your instrument—learn how to "play" it in the zone of peak performance.

Maximize Your Performance

One of the goals of yoga is to attain a state of oneness with the universe. Surprisingly, this goal has endless practical applications. When your mind and body are one, and one with the power of the universe, the sense of tranquillity and control you can achieve makes everything clearer and simpler. Everything you do will be affected. Do you have a big presentation at work? You are calm, confident, and empowered. Do you have a championship tennis match? You are strong, flexible, buoyant, and the ball seems to go exactly where you will it to go. Do you have a really difficult test? Your mind is so uncluttered that all your studying comes back to you effortlessly.

Of course, such power doesn't come easily. A week of sitting in the lotus position for five minutes a day won't be enough to send you permanently into "the zone." Yoga is a process. Your body and your mind need to learn new habits and a new way to communicate with each other. But if you're persistent and follow the yoga path, you'll quickly perceive the changes blessing your life. You'll feel peace of mind, even the ecstasy of oneness with the life force. And you will be in the best shape you've ever been in, too.

So what are you waiting for?

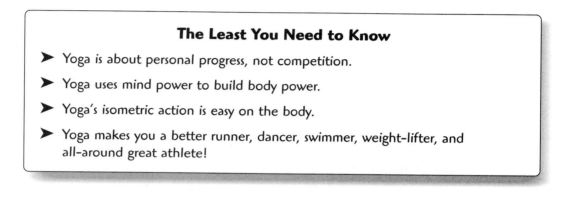

The Least You Need to Know

➤ Yoga is about personal progress, not competition.

➤ Yoga uses mind power to build body power.

➤ Yoga's isometric action is easy on the body.

➤ Yoga makes you a better runner, dancer, swimmer, weight-lifter, and all-around great athlete!

Chapter 3

How Comfortable Are You in Your Body?

In This Chapter

➤ A self-test for the yoga-challenged

➤ Understanding how your body works

➤ Using yoga to learn to trust your body

You know the types who are comfortable in their bodies. You've seen them gliding through life looking ready for anything. They don't slouch or slump or hunch over. They don't have flawless bodies. (Nobody does.) But they don't seem to mind! They look like they feel great in their own skin, no matter what shape or size they happen to be.

Are you comfortable in *your* body? Are standing, sitting, and lying down easy, or do you feel your clothes binding, your stomach sagging, your back aching, and your knees cracking? Can you spring up from a sitting position on the floor like a child, or is hoisting yourself to a stand always accompanied by grunts, long sighs, and various strange popping noises from assorted joints?

The truth of the matter is that most of us aren't comfortable in our bodies. Why? Two reasons: We don't maintain them as well as we might, and we are convinced, for any number of reasons, that we *should* look and feel different than we do. Fitness expert Jack LaLanne once said that if more people treated their bodies with the same care and upkeep they give to their most precious possessions (their houses and their cars), everyone would be fitter and healthier. Isn't a little maintenance worth the effort?

And what about maintenance on your body image? That could probably use a little ratcheting, too.

A Self-Test for the Yoga-Challenged

Are you yoga-challenged? In other words, are you so far out of touch with your body that yoga seems like an impossibility? Take this test to find out how in tune you are with your body. Choose the one best answer for each question.

1. The longest amount of time I can sit on the floor without feeling some sort of pain and discomfort is ...

   a. Thirty minutes or longer.

   b. Fifteen minutes, max.

   c. Maybe two minutes.

   d. Why the heck would I want to sit on the floor? That's why they invented the couch.

2. My back ...

   a. Never hurts.

   b. Hurts 24 hours a day.

   c. Hurts after I've been sitting for too long.

   d. Hurts when I don't exercise regularly.

3. My coccyx is ...

   a. The vertebrae at the base of my neck.

   b. My kneecap.

   c. A small, triangular bone at the base of my spine.

   d. I'm quite sure I don't have a coccyx!

4. I get sick (cold, flu, gastroenteritis, etc.) or injured (sprained ankle, twisted knee, back goes out, etc.) at least ...

   a. Once a year.

   b. Once every few months.

   c. Once every few weeks.

   d. I hardly ever get sick or injured.

5. My vision is ...

   a. Excellent (20/20 or better).

   b. Pretty good. I have glasses or contacts, but my prescription isn't a very strong one.

    c. Terrible. I can't see well at all without my glasses or contacts.

    d. I'm sorry, I couldn't quite make out the question. It's too blurry.

6. Whenever I feel a cold coming on, the first thing I do is …

    a. Push fluids, get more sleep, go in late to work, and drag myself through the day.

    b. Try to talk myself out of it or ignore it. I don't have time to get sick!

    c. Go to work, but whine and complain that I'm getting sick while sneezing and coughing all over my co-workers.

    d. Rest, bundle up on the couch with some herbal tea with lemon and honey, increase my vitamin C intake, and stay home so I can get better.

7. The difference between tendons and ligaments is …

    a. Tendons connect muscles to bones, while ligaments connect bones to bones or hold organs in place.

    b. Tendons connect bones to bones or hold organs in place, while ligaments connect muscles to bones.

    c. Tendons and ligaments are those things I'm always pulling and tearing, after which my doctor says, "There's nothing I can do."

    d. Huh?

8. The way I feel about my body can best be described as follows …

    a. I dislike certain parts of my body, but other parts are pleasing. I'm good at disguising my faults with my clothing.

    b. My body is okay, but I don't pay much attention to it.

    c. I love my body. I think it's beautiful, and it feels good to be in it. I take good care of it so it will stay that way.

    d. I practically have a heart attack every time I look in the mirror, so I just don't look in the mirror.

9. I can …

    a. Bend down and touch my toes easily.

    b. Bend down and touch my knees easily.

    c. Fold completely in half, bending forward, hugging my calves with my arms, and resting my head and entire upper body against my legs.

    d. Look down and almost see my feet.

10. My muscles are visible …

    a. In a lot of places if I flex. I can see the line of my calf muscle if I stand on my toes, and I can see my biceps and triceps if I flex my arm.

b. All the time. I can see my thigh muscles, calf muscles, biceps, triceps, deltoids, and abdominal muscles, even without flexing them. I am truly buff!

c. Possibly on an x-ray—that is, if x-rays showed muscles.

d. Every now and then. Especially when I'm at a lower weight, I can see something that looks a little bit like muscle, but mostly I just see smooth, rounded surfaces with some bumpy cellulite here and there.

Now score your test by giving yourself the correct number of points, as indicated below, for each answer. For example, for each question you answered with an a, give yourself three points. For each b, you get two points. Add up your points, and then check the following section to see what your score means.

a. 3

b. 2

c. 1

d. 0

Your score: _____

What Your Body Is Telling You, and Whether It's Good News

So, how'd you do on the quiz?

If you scored 25 to 30 points: Are you already a *yogi* and just reading this book for fun? You have a wonderful awareness of your body. If you aren't doing yoga, you'll probably love it.

If you scored 16 to 24 points: There are a few things you don't like about your body, but at least you pay attention to it. As you work through yoga's exercises and meditations, your bad habits will eventually disappear on their own. You won't need willpower, because treating your body well will feel so good!

If you scored 8 to 15 points: Yoga can help you become more aware of your body and improve your self-image. You'll discover feelings, muscles, positions, and energy you never imagined you had. If you don't pay attention to your body, it will break down faster, and you don't want that!

If you scored 0 to 7 points: Talk about somebody who needs yoga! You're barely aware of your body at all, either because you ignore it or because you dislike it so much that you want nothing to do with it. Yoga can gently coax you into a new relationship with your body—one based on respect and appreciation.

Most of us have many illusions about our bodies. Unfortunately, these illusions affect not only our feelings about our physical appearance, but also our self-esteem and our relations with others. Be aware that the following italicized statements about your body are *not true:*

➤ *Your body is without consciousness, and your mind is separate from your body.* **Not so.** Many of your organs and tissues have properties similar to your brain, sending out messages, receiving information, reacting accordingly, and letting you know when you're being abusive or kind to your body. Your entire body is awake, alive, and aware.

➤ *You can't change your body.* **Of course you can!** Not only can you change your body profoundly through your actions and thoughts, but your body continuously changes itself: All your cells are replaced every five years. Your body is supremely mutable.

➤ *Your body is solid.* **It only looks that way.** Actually, at the atomic level, your body consists of vibrating atoms with lots of space in between. You are more energy than matter!

➤ *Bodies are a curse.* **Not at all!** Bodies are an opportunity and a tool through which the inner soul can be discovered.

➤ *I am a victim of genetics.* **You don't have to be a victim.** Genetics only reveal the make and model of your body. What you do with that body and that mind and how you care for them can be as powerful as your genes.

➤ *People judge you by your body, first and foremost.* **No they don't, even when they think they do.** Your self-concept is a powerful force that emanates from you and influences others more than you might think.

Ouch!

Stop punishing yourself! Hating your body is unnatural; why not give yoga a try? The postures will improve your health, and yoga's meditation will help your mind feel more benevolent toward your body. Life is too short to ignore or berate the primary mechanism that houses your soul.

The Shape You Are In

To know your body is to love your body, with all its unique characteristics. Whether you tend to be muscular, curvy, slim, or some combination, look around and you'll see others with many of the same qualities—and different physical characteristics of all kinds, too.

But knowing your body type can do more than make you feel satisfied that there are plenty of other people who have a similar shape. Your body type can give you clues to what types of yoga poses will come more easily to you, and what types of poses might be more challenging and balancing for your body type.

(Keep in mind as you read the descriptions for each of the body types that any body type can belong to either men or women.)

Love your body, whether you're an ectomorph, en-domorph, or mesomorph. It takes all kinds to make a world!

Ectomorph   Endomorph   Mesomorph

The Slim Ectomorph

The ectomorph body type tends to be tall and slender with narrow shoulders and hips, long limbs, relatively low body fat, and underdeveloped muscles. Although the stereotypical ectomorph is slender because of a tendency to have a lower muscle mass, ectomorphs can develop a high fat-to-muscle ratio if they don't get enough exercise.

Luckily, exercise is easy for ectomorphs, who tend to be highly energetic and who, when in shape, can bounce effortlessly through a high-impact aerobics class followed by a three-mile run. Good luck keeping up with an ectomorph's pace. Unless you are also an ectomorph, it won't be easy.

Aerobic activity, however, while healthy in moderation, isn't as important for ecto-morphs as developing those muscles. Everyone needs cardiovascular exercise, but ec-tomorphs may tend to overdo this type of activity because it comes so easily. Not so easy for ectomorphs is weight training.

Yoga is great for ectomorphs because it can help to slow that frantic pace they tend to maintain. Yoga is also a weight-bearing activity, so it is the perfect, gentle way to in-troduce ectomorphs to their own muscles. Because many yoga poses lift, hold, and/or balance the body's own weight, yoga provides ectomorphs with the muscle-developing and strength-building exercise their body type requires to maintain a physical fitness equilibrium.

Your ectomorph summary:

➤ Narrow shoulders and hips

➤ Long limbs

➤ Low body-fat to muscle-mass ratio

➤ High energy

➤ Benefits from yoga poses that are calming and poses that develop muscle strength

The Curvaceous Endomorph

The endomorph is the classic Rubenesque figure: all curves and rounded surfaces. Endomorphs aren't automatically overweight, but they do tend to have a higher fat-to-muscle ratio than the other body types, accumulating fat on the abdomen, buttocks, hips, and thighs.

They tend to be pear-shaped, with narrower shoulders and wider hips than ectomorphs.

Endomorphs have slower metabolisms and may seem more languid or serene than the energetic and active ectomorph. This natural tendency, when not countered with regular activity, may result in a sedentary lifestyle, something that isn't healthy for anyone. Endomorphs burn fat more slowly, and it takes more steady, low-intensity aerobic exercise for them to burn fat than it would for an ectomorph, making exercise crucial to maintaining a healthy weight.

Yoga is perfect for endomorphs, too. Many yoga exercises are low-intensity aerobic exercises that burn fat. Endomorphs might want to pay particular attention to *vinyasa,* such as the sun salutation (see Chapter 16, "A Continuous Flow"), groups of yoga poses strung together with coordinated breathing patterns. These pose series are just what the endomorph needs to burn off any extra fat that develops and impart the energy some endomorphs have difficulty generating.

Endomorphs also tend to have a naturally strong lower body, but the endomorph's upper body often needs development. Many yoga exercises involve lifting and holding body weight with the upper body. These poses will help the endomorph to develop a more balanced body.

Know Your Sanskrit

Vinyasa is a steady flow of connected yoga *asanas* linked with breathwork in a continuous movement. It is a dynamic form of yoga.

Your endomorph summary:

➤ Narrow shoulders and wide hips

➤ High body-fat to muscle-mass ratio

➤ Strong lower body

➤ A relaxed disposition, sometimes bordering on inactive

➤ Benefits from an aerobic series of yoga poses like the sun salutation, and poses that build upper body strength

The Muscular Mesomorph

The mesomorph develops muscle mass easily and has a high muscle-mass-to-body-fat ratio. Mesomorphs tend to accumulate fat around the waist, triceps, and back, but mesomorphs who get physical activity have well-developed muscles. It doesn't take much for a mesomorph to sport washboard abs, cut triceps, or an impressively muscled back.

Strength is the mesomorph's forte, so the weight-bearing aspect of yoga makes the mesomorph feel right at home. Too much weight-bearing exercise can actually bulk up a mesomorph too much.

Mesomorphs tend to be more easily motivated than endomorphas, and may feel right at home with the weight-bearing yoga poses, but stretching is another matter. Those tight mesomorph muscles don't tend to be particularly flexible.

Yoga to the rescue! Yoga is perhaps *the* best exercise for developing long, strong, flexible muscles. The aerobic aspect of yoga is also helpful for mesomorphs, since their tendency to develop fat around the middle may put them at greater risk for heart disease.

A Yoga Minute

The classic muscle-bound weight-lifter tends to be a mesomorph. Mesomorphs who don't want to look too bulky should limit weight-bearing activities to those who use lighter weights and more repetitions.

Your mesomorph summary:

➤ Muscular upper and lower body

➤ High muscle-mass-to-body-fat ratio

➤ Accumulates fat around the middle

➤ An easily motivated disposition

➤ Benefits from moderately aerobic yoga poses and poses that lengthen and increase the flexibility of muscles

Your Body and Yoga 101

Yoga can help you optimize the particular physical body you've been given, but your physical makeup isn't the whole picture. You are also animated by energy. Your cultural background determines the way you may see or understand your body in all its layers and complexities, and your own personal level of confidence and trust in your own body can teach you even more about the complex package otherwise known as you.

Your Personal Energy Cycle

No matter how in touch or out of touch you are with your body, everyone has energy cycles. You know, even without consciously knowing, when your energy levels fluctuate. Sometimes your energy peaks, sometimes it lags. Sometimes you wake up ready to go-go-go, and sometimes you can barely pull yourself out of bed. Energy cycles can be affected by increased activity, over- or undereating, or too little sleep. Your monthly cycles, the weather, lunar cycles, and your health, diet, and regular level of exercise can all have an effect, too.

Just as people have different body types, they have different energy patterns. Maybe you tend to wake up ready to take on the world, but by nighttime, you can't wait to crawl into bed. Or maybe you don't want to see another human face before 10 A.M., but at midnight, you are ready to rock. While individual energy fluctuations can be a matter of habit (you can accustom yourself to working the night shift, for example), working with your natural energy flow will make yoga easier and more enjoyable, and a regular yoga practice will smooth out your natural energy flow.

A Yoga Minute

Are you a night owl or a lark? Night owls typically enjoy energy peaks about two hours later in the day than larks, who are the classic "morning people." Typical larks enjoy the morning and a good breakfast and feel most alert and creative early in the day, preferring to retire early. Night owls often dislike eating breakfast and enjoy their peak later in the day, preferring to stay up late and sleep in.

When energy shoots up or plummets too suddenly, we are left feeling exhausted, out of balance, even confused. That sudden five-story drop on the roller coaster may be thrilling for a few seconds, but those nice, smooth hills and valleys are a lot less jarring on your system. Yoga helps your energy cycles flow smoothly. Instead of super highs and abysmal lows, you can enjoy a steady stream of energy, like an exhalation of air you control by the size of the opening of your lips and the force of your exhalation.

With the regular practice of yoga, energy lows blend into energy highs, and the highs flow easily into the lows. Yoga helps you get in touch with and pay closer attention to these cycles as it softens the transitions between them, making you feel more even and balanced all day and all night.

The Muscle and Bone Connection

If we go skin deeper, we get to your bones and muscles. Yoga postures make more sense if you know a little bit about how your body works. Your particular physical challenges will also become more specific to you if you understand your anatomy.

Your skeleton is your frame. It supports your fat, muscles, and organs. It contains 206 bones. Connecting the muscles to the bones are tendons. Muscles help you bend your joints and perform all sorts of tasks. Strong muscles go a long way toward supporting your frame, making it easier to achieve good posture. Think about how effortlessly infants curl up and raise their toes to their mouth. Your back and spine are completely loose before you learn to walk. Once walking begins, the spine tightens and flexibility diminishes and diminishes and … Yoga is the caretaker of the spine, lengthening and extending it to release the energy that runs through this neural superhighway.

The Western anatomical model of the human body's musculoskeletal and nervous systems (left) is complemented by yoga's seven energy centers, called chakras *(right), which store and release* prana, *the life force.*

Eastern Body, Western Body

Is your body different than the body of someone from a different part of the world? Of course not, but different cultures have different theories about the body. The concept that the body and the mind are one is an easy concept for the Easterner. The physical body is merely one of several "bodies." It's a temple to house the spirit but should be well-tended and rigorously cared for because of the importance of what it holds. The *astral* body is the vehicle of the spirit and is maintained through breathing, meditation, and concentration. The *causal* body is the place where the spirit works. The ego is absent from the causal body, and the spirit can know its true potential here. Ideally, the spirit transcends all bodies and becomes pure consciousness, an individual expression of the divine. To the traditional Easterner, the mind/body is sacred, not to be abused, but to be used as a vehicle for the spirit's expression, which results, finally, in enlightenment.

On the other side of the spectrum is the Westerner. Traditionally, the Westerner sees one part of the self at a time. The body is the body. Healthy food keeps it running, and exercise keeps it strong. End of story. Then there is the mind. The mind is the source of intelligence and thought. Activities that stimulate the mind, from philosophical conversations to crossword puzzles, keep the mind active. End of story. Then there is the spirit. The spirit might be nurtured and maintained by going to church or by a personal philosophy or spirituality. In many, the spirit is ignored. End of story.

Westerners have certainly survived—and thrived. So why should we change a system that works? Because it keeps us off balance. Westerners are movers and shakers, yet many of us exist on the edge of health and sanity, surviving on caffeine, nicotine, and sugar, wracked by stress and saddled with materialism, ego, desire, and greed. We need something to even us out, calm us down, and get us in touch with ourselves again. Don't believe that this will slow you down or make you less effective. Integrating mind, body, and spirit can only make you a better and more effective, productive person—Westerner or Easterner.

Wise Yogi Tells Us

Moderation is the wisest, most peace-inspiring course. Nothing should be so important that it must be had in excess, and nothing should be so unimportant that it must be utterly denied.

Do You Trust Your Body?

Maybe you've never thought of your body in terms of something you should or shouldn't trust, but you have an intimate relationship with your body. It's your vehicle for communicating with the world. Do you trust your body? How many of the following statements do you agree with?

➤ "When I get a craving, I can't control my eating. I'll eat an entire quart of ice cream, a huge steak, a pound of chocolate, candy, a whole pizza, and a pie. I can't stop myself."

➤ "I'm accident-prone, especially when I play sports or exercise. I always twist an ankle, jam a thumb, or injure myself in some other way."

➤ "I always get sick just when an important event is about to happen. My body betrays me when I need it most!"

➤ "I don't know what to think about myself, because what I see in the mirror is totally different than how other people describe me."

➤ "I'm uncomfortable in most of my clothes."

If you agreed with any of these statements, you have problems trusting your body. Your body is not your enemy, and it's not a stranger. While you may need professional help to cure an eating disorder, chronic illness, or negative self-image (you'll want to enlist the aid of a licensed healthcare professional as well as a yoga instructor!), the wonderful thing about yoga is that it reacquaints you with your physical self. You'll get to know your body like never before, and you'll even learn to make peace with your body, enjoy your body, *like* your body.

Your body will begin to respond the way you intend. You'll know what your body is going to do. You'll be paying attention. You'll have more control over your physical being and mental state, so you'll be injured less, be more sure about what you think, be in better control of what you do, and be more self-confident.

The Least You Need to Know

➤ Yoga helps you feel better in your body.

➤ Body awareness is an important part of practicing yoga.

➤ The ectomorph body type tends to be tall, thin, and energetic; the endomorph body type tends to be curvy with wide hips and a more relaxed temperament; the mesomorph body type tends to be strong with well-developed muscles and an even temperament.

➤ The more you pay attention to and learn your own personal anatomy, energy cycles, and body image issues, the more you will integrate your mind and body for greater confidence and self-control.

➤ Yoga can help you learn to trust your body.

Chapter 4

Yoga Mind Power: Go with the Flow

In This Chapter

➤ Finding peace in a stressful world

➤ What meditation teaches us

➤ Reaching the yoga zone of flow

➤ Flow in an actual yoga pose

Life is not a war, it's not a contest, and it's not a race. Life is *being*. Yoga helps you see this truth and live it each moment. The need to name, label, evaluate, and analyze everything we come into contact with can be debilitating to the spirit. Yoga teaches you to look without classifying, to listen without judging, to feel without losing control, to learn without assuming you already know—simply, to be.

Everything is subjective. Realizing this will help bring peace to your busily categorizing mind and help you see the truth in difficult situations, people, and even yourself. Labels make perception seem easy, but perception isn't easy, so banish the labels and look harder and closer at yourself and the world. Let yoga show you how.

A Fight-or-Flight World

There's no doubt about it—we live in a stressful world! The human animal has a specific way to deal with stress, and it's called the *fight-or-flight response*. When confronted with a stressful situation, your adrenaline starts pumping. Your muscles tense. Your senses heighten. In essence, your body becomes primed to deal with the stress in two ways: either fight with the utmost energy and strength, or get away as fast as possible. How can fight or flight help you? It gives you energy. It gives you a quick reaction time. Your mind is sharper and clearer. If you recognize all this and work with your body, your experience of a stressful situation—say, presenting a new product line at work or teaching a class to a new group of students—will be vibrant and exciting.

The problem with the fight-or-flight response comes when it's engaged too often. Bodies can take only much stress, and if your body and mind are forced into a constant elevated state of stimulation, muscle tension, and excess energy, you're bound to break down. Maybe you'll get sick, collapse from exhaustion, or just plain lose your ability to communicate so that others can understand you. The problem with our world is that it constantly bombards us with stressful situations. What's more, our culture rewards those who take on the most stress. Who do you admire more—your colleagues who are always taking on projects and coming up with new ideas, working late every night, and helping everyone else who gets behind? Or the colleagues who relax at their desks talking on the phone, leave at five with overflowing in-boxes, and never seem in a hurry to get anything done?

We want the overachievers on our team: the high-powered, assertive, I-can-do-anything types. With that kind of pressure, it's no wonder we're all under so much stress.

Enter yoga! In a fight-or-flight world, yoga is like a daily trip to the spa. Not only will it relax you and calm your mind, it can fine-tune the fight-or-flight response. With yoga, you learn to clear your mind and listen. You learn to focus, concentrate, and tune in. Obstacles that confuse us and prohibit us from seeing clearly are gently washed away with yoga. When the fight-or-flight response kicks in, the yoga practitioner can channel it so that it's as productive as possible. When your muscles tense, you're aware of them and can direct their energy to stand straighter, move more quickly, and react more deftly. As your senses heighten and your thinking sharpens, you'll see how to clear your mind of everything but the task at hand. Answers will come to you. The perfect combination of words will flow effortlessly from your mouth. You'll be able to perceive your situation clearly—the motivations of others, your position in the circumstances, and what should be done. Panic is replaced by confidence.

Yoga isn't magic. It doesn't turn you into someone you aren't—but yoga is the key to making the fight-or-flight response work for you, because it gives you control over your physical and mental responses to this instinct.

Concentration, Relaxation, Meditation

Meditation is an important part of yoga. But maybe you aren't interested in meditating. That's fine—just practice the *asanas*. Chances are, however, that the more you progress through the *asanas*, the more interested you'll become in meditation. Meditation can do wonderful things for your mind and your body.

Perhaps you aren't sure what meditation is. Really, it's a simple concept. Meditation is the process of attaining total awareness through the cessation of thought. You begin by relaxing. You concentrate on relaxing. Perhaps you feel like a wave relaxing into the ocean, because that's what you are. You are a part of the universe the way a wave is part of the ocean. In fact, repetition of the *mantra Om* even sounds like waves on the shore. Soon your thought waves decrease and become still. The wise Indian sage Patanjali said, "Yoga is the cessation of the fluctuations of the mind." We say "Still waters run deep."

As you let your mind relax, notice the thoughts that come to you. Acknowledge them, then let them go. This is difficult at first. We are so used to having busy minds. Especially if you've never meditated before, you may find it virtually impossible to stop following and obsessing over the thoughts racing through your mind. You may think about chores you should be doing, a problem at work, a fight you had with your spouse or child, what to make for dinner, or what you plan to do that weekend. We are conditioned to believe that every minute should count and that we should always be getting as much done as possible. But yoga disagrees with this notion. Yoga says that the mind needs to be stilled occasionally to keep it working at peak efficiency. Face it: You wouldn't leave all the appliances on in your house all day long every day and expect them to work properly for a long period of time. Things would go haywire, burn out, blow out, blow up, or break down.

A Yoga Minute

Patanjali was an Indian sage who, thousands of years ago, wrote a text called the *Yoga Sutra*, which recorded concepts that had been passed down orally for many years. This influential text, which consists of a series of aphorisms about how to practice yoga, has helped to define the modern practice of yoga.

Ouch!

Even meditation can be counterproductive. Although you probably won't pull a muscle while meditating, it's possible to stay stressed, or even to become more stressed, in your efforts to relax! Don't think. Don't worry that you aren't meditating correctly. Feel your body, feel your breathing, and feel who you are. Let your thoughts flow through your mind like pictures on a movie screen, flickering and passing on. Gently, lovingly, let each thought go. Ahhhh!

So why should your mind be any different? It isn't a perpetual motion machine. If you don't learn how to calm and still your mind, it's bound to need some loving care and maintenance. We're not saying that if you don't meditate, you'll go nuts (though it's possible!). What we're saying is that a neglected mind is one that doesn't work as well as it could. Meditation is mental maintenance. Teaching yourself how to relax your mind and release it from the stress of thought for a short period each day keeps it clear and clean. You'll think better. You'll see more accurately and with more insight. You'll be able to concentrate and focus on things like never before. You'll be able to truly relax. In fact, you'll probably be amazed at the mind power you never knew you had.

From Full Mind to Mindfulness

What is stillness? Simply a lack of movement? As you move through your daily life, stillness would probably not be an adjective you would use to describe your mental state. You are busy, you have responsibilities, and you are good at what you do. This takes a full mind, a mind always thinking about what to do next. A mind prepared to deal with conflict. A mind ready to tackle anything, whether it's a toddler's temper tantrum or capturing a multimillion-dollar account for your company. Who has time for stillness when you've got so much to *do?*

You do, because stillness will take your full mind; empty it out; give it a good, thorough cleaning; and transform it into a mindful mind. What does that mean? A mindful mind is like a mirror that is meticulously polished. It reflects what is really there and nothing else. When you become mindful, you learn to suspend everything you believe about yourself, others, and the world. Your limits, your shortcomings, your fears, what people have told you that you can and can't do—all these are put on hold. What's left is the real you, and your possibilities are limitless. Mindfulness takes courage. It can be scary to look at the real you. But if you take a good look, you'll have new power. You'll understand who you are like never before.

And, as your self-concept expands, so will your concept of the world. Everything is within your grasp. Yet you aren't grasping—you're simply living, achieving, and being the best person you can possibly be. Have you heard the phrase "optimize your hard drive"? That's not just for your personal computer. Yoga optimizes the hard drive in your head! This involves extending your meditation to your daily life. Once you've made meditation a part of your life, you can gradually learn to carry its principles with you throughout your day. When negative feelings arise, gently push them away as if they were balloons. Look at them, note them, acknowledge them, and then let go of the string. If people are unkind, unfair, or judgmental of you, you can learn to gently push these balloons away, too.

Meditation in daily life means remembering the peace and stillness you've learned to achieve during regular meditation, then finding that peace and stillness throughout the day. The real you will shine through best when you're in touch with this inner peace.

Wise Yogi Tells Us

To help yourself meditate, think of all the definitions of yourself you know. "I am a teacher." "I am a father." "I am bad at math." "I am talented." "I am shy." "I am lazy." "I am well-meaning." "I am jealous." Now pretend these definitions are untrue. Just pretend. Then look beyond. What's left is the real you, and you may be surprised at what you see. Surprised and pleased, as if you've met an old friend you haven't seen in years ... maybe even in lifetimes!

Relax Past Your Boundaries

What are your boundaries? We all have them, and they are all branches of *avidya,* or our false perceptions of life and of ourselves. Boundaries limit us from the truth and from our potential. Some of the boundaries we impose upon ourselves are known as *asmita,* or ego; *raga,* or attachment; *dvesha,* or rejection; and *abhinivesha,* or the survival instinct.

Know Your Sanskrit

Avidya (pronounced *ah-VEE-dyah*) is the word for incorrect comprehension. The opposite of *avidya* is **vidya** (*VEE-dyah*), correct understanding. *Avidya* inhibits our perception in many ways—through automatic, learned responses; dependency on habits; and negative self-talk. *Avidya* is like a cloud in front of the sun. Learning to recognize *avidya* and dispel it is one of the goals of yoga. **Asmita** (*ah-SMEE-tah*) is the ego, **raga** (*RAH-gah*) is attachment, and **dvesha** (*DVEH-shah*) is rejection.

Ego is a boundary difficult for most Westerners to avoid. Your ego is what gives you a sense of who you are to the world. To say, "I am the smartest one in this class," is ego. To say, "I have to win this game," is ego. To say, "I am beautiful," or "I am right," or even "I am good at my job," is ego. To most Westerners, some expression of ego seems natural and even productive. Why not be proud of what you do, how you look, or what you've accomplished? You certainly should be proud of who you are. But *asmita* means being proud of the wrong things—the things that limit you, such as material possessions, physical appearance, beating out someone, or being the best, which implies you're better than others.

Deep inside, you're a jewel. You're a beautiful soul that's part of a beautiful universe. Getting caught up in the petty and nonlasting aspects of life can only hold you back from your true potential. Maybe you still think you have to be competitive to "win," but yoga can help you to see winning in a new, more fulfilling light.

Attachment is related to ego and involves desire. Do you know what it's like to want a cookie or a piece of cake, not because you're truly hungry but just because you want the pleasure? The desire for pleasure can overcome you, and you can be fiercely single-minded until you get what you want. If you've experienced this feeling, then you know what *raga* is. Attachment also involves material possessions—that sort of "fever" you get when you see something you really want. It can consume your entire mind—the desire for that new dress, stereo system, or hot red sports car. Attachment to any material possessions, sensual sensations, addictions, desires, or even an obsessive attachment to another person is a boundary that holds you back from truth and the true knowledge of yourself. Attachment gets in the way of who you really are.

Rejection is like the opposite of attachment and is called *dvesha*. Your spouse left you, so you refuse to get involved in a relationship again. You were thrown from a horse, so you refuse to ride. You were in a car accident, so you vow never to drive another car. All these are *dvesha*. Rejecting experiences, people, or thoughts that have caused you pain in the past blocks you from the future. But *dvesha* needn't be so drastic, and we all experience it. You refuse to try okra because you think it will taste unpleasant. You don't go to a party because you know the social interactions will be stressful and you just don't have the energy. This isn't to say that you can't make the decision not to do certain things, but when you reject things out of a fear of discomfort, pain, or inconvenience, rather than rejecting things simply because you don't want or need them, then *dvesha* has become a stumbling block in your life.

The final obstacle is the survival instinct, or *abhinivesha*. This instinct may seem to be a positive one at first, but it is actually a stumbling block between you and enlightenment. This intense desire to remain alive is related to the fear of death (although they aren't the same). You probably want to remain you. You may fear death, but you also enjoy your life (for the most part) and so fear any kind of change in your existence. Enlightenment, involving release from the material world and tangible existence, is both mysterious and scary. Does enlightenment mean that life as we know it will cease? We are animals, after all. Our instincts are for self-preservation. Moving beyond our instinctual natures into our spiritual selves isn't easy.

Wise Yogi Tells Us

"Heart breathing" is a technique that can be very renewing. Sit comfortably. Close your eyes. Notice your breathing, but don't try to control it. Feel your chest expanding and contracting. Now imagine the breath is flowing out of your heart with each exhalation and pouring into your heart with each inhalation. Don't think about anything. Just feel the breath flowing in and out of your heart. Imagine the breath is pure love. Do this for 5 to 10 minutes, then slowly open your eyes, get up, and move on. Remember the feeling throughout your day. Then do it again tomorrow!

Yoga helps dispel *abhinivesha* (the survival instinct), as well as the other aspects of *avidya* (incorrect comprehension) that cloud our perception and inhibit our growth.

Sure, you'll probably always have occasional bouts of ego, attachment, rejection, and the instinct to cling to your material existence. You are only human—and not *only* human, but deeply, magnificently human. Through yoga, you can become even more deeply connected to your true humanity. You can learn to recognize your incorrect comprehension for what it is, then you can blow out the incarnations of your incorrect comprehension like matches. No more delusions!

Yoga helps you relax, think more clearly, and see the inner you that is a part of the universe and all that is good. Yoga helps reveal *avidya* for the impostor it is. And if you can perceive the stumbling blocks in your path clearly and without doubt, you can confidently step around them.

Know Your Sanskrit

Abhinivesha (*ah-bhee-nee-VEH-shah*) is the survival instinct or thirst for life. It is the desire to exist and so becomes an obstacle toward enlightenment, which is existence but beyond the personal existence to which unenlightened individuals cling.

Find the Zone—and Move In!

We've already talked about the *zone*. The zone is that place you go when your skill is suddenly heightened, your mind is sharp, and you can do no wrong. Athletes know about the zone. When an athlete is in the zone, he or she has reached peak perform-ance. The mind is thinking quickly, sharply, and accurately. Success is effortless.

Ouch!

Do not sit awkwardly during meditation. Sitting slumped over with a crooked spine, or sitting in a position too advanced for you, can cause injury to your body, as well as frustration. It's impossible to relax deeply into your meditation if your body is strained or in pain. So stay within your physical limits while medi-tating and concentrate on your mind instead.

Artists know about the zone. It's the place where noth-ing else exists but the task at hand. A painting seems to paint itself. The words to a novel flow effortlessly. The sculpture emerges, the actor becomes the charac-ter, and the dancer becomes one with the dance.

Students know about the zone. It's that rare time when the answers to a test are obvious to you, and all the information you've studied seems immediately available. Your brain exceeds itself, the words to an essay write themselves, and the meanings to formulas suddenly become clear.

Another word for the zone in contemporary culture is *flow*. Anyone can achieve flow, but some achieve it more often than others. You have flow when you be-come completely absorbed in what you're doing. Time seems to stop, nothing else exists, and you become one with your work. During flow, you can accomplish things you never thought you could.

Wouldn't it be nice to achieve flow whenever you wanted—to move into the zone and live there all the time? For most, flow comes and goes, seemingly ac-cording to its own whim. But for the experienced yoga practitioner, the zone is a place to go whenever you choose. Because yoga uses control of the body to still the mind and control of the mind to manipulate the body, body and mind become integrated not only with each other, but also with the external world. If you're one with your work, your art, or your sport, you've achieved flow. You're in the zone.

Yoga is like a key to the secret door into the zone. Open it, and you'll live beyond your limits, finding new productivity, creativity, efficiency, and true delight.

Go with the Flow Right Here, Right Now

It's fine to read all about getting into the zone, but how do you actually get there? By cultivating mindful awareness and focus.

Would you like to try it? Let's take a basic yoga pose, called the cobra pose (*Bhujan-gasana,* in Sanskrit), and practice getting into and out of it. Look at the following pic-ture of the pose and read through the step-by-step instructions before you try it. Make sure you are wearing comfortable clothes that don't constrict your movement. Place a towel, blanket, or mat on the floor.

Before you jump into the pose ...

1. Let's sit for a moment. Sit comfortably on the floor and breathe. Don't worry about breathing deeply. Just notice your breath. Give your breath your full at-tention. You can probably "hear" lots of thoughts rattling around in your mind, somewhere behind the sound of your breathing. Note them, but don't let them engage you. Back to the breath.

2. After you've been sitting for a minute or two with your mind focused on your breath, move into a lying-down position on your stomach. But don't just move thoughtlessly. As you move, really pay attention. Keep your mind centered on how you feel, on how your body moves, on which parts are going where as you come down to the floor. Your body is all that matters right now, and a great yoga pose like this deserves all your concentration. With every step of this pose, keep pulling your focus back to your body; the way the pose feels; the way you move and breathe as you get into, hold, and get out of the pose. You are practic-ing mindfulness. You are in flow training.

The cobra pose.

43

a. Lie on your stomach, flat on the floor, with your heels and toes together. Place your hands on the floor on either side of your chest. Your face should be resting against the floor.

b. Inhale, and lift your forehead, then chin, then shoulders, and then chest off the floor. Keep your hips pressed against the floor and your elbows bent, shoulders down and away from your ears.

c. Look upward and take a few slow, deep breaths. Then try sticking out your tongue and opening your mouth wide, to help release your face. Finally, slowly come back down and return to the starting position.

d. To test the strength of your spine, lift your palms off the floor, as you see in the lower figure in the drawing. See how much of your body comes down—if it's a lot, your arms are doing too much of the work. Focus on the spine instead. The emphasis of cobra pose is to strengthen the spine.

e. Now, slowly push yourself out of cobra by pushing up with your hands and sitting back on your heels. Rest your forehead on the floor and relax, giving your spine a chance to stretch in the opposite direction. This position is called child's pose.

3. Stay in this last position for a few minutes.

How was it? Did you stay focused on your body, your movements, how the pose felt? Are you still focused on your body? As you rest in this ending position, let your body feel the aftereffects of the cobra pose. What do you notice? How does your mind feel? At any point during the process, do all those clattering thoughts in the back of your mind recede? Do they stop clattering altogether?

A Yoga Minute

Yoga is truly a mind/body exercise. The mind focuses on the body, the body responds to the mind. The two are partners in the process, and your whole being becomes more fully integrated.

Maybe you got a little taste of flow during this exercise. Maybe you didn't. But if you practice yoga every day with this kind of attention, eventually you'll experience flow. You have it in you.

Practicing yoga poses is a kind of meditation itself. With this approach, you can train your mind to be flow-ready. It will happen more and more. You'll finally know what it's like to be yourself!

Release Your Inner Delight

Joy, bliss, ecstasy—whatever you want to call it—is yoga's big payoff. Maybe you consider yourself a happy person, or maybe you suffer from depression. Maybe you had a happy childhood, or maybe you've been hurt in the past. It doesn't matter: No matter who you are, no matter what has happened to you in your life, you have the capacity for joy. Deep inside you, bliss waits for you to find it. Yoga will ferret out that joy with relentless persistence. Through yoga, you can find that joy and release it.

But make no mistake: It isn't easy to release your inner delight. A body that's undisciplined, weak, and lazy saps all your inner energy to keep it maintained. A mind fraught with chaotic thought is too absorbed on the surface level to delve deep enough to find inner joy. But with persistent yoga practice, the body becomes strong, controlled, flexible, and disciplined. The mind becomes quiet, calm, and tranquil. A restless body that at one time struggled to maintain the lotus position for an extended period and a mind that regularly wandered without purpose now both respond with focus and commitment.

Wise Yogi Tells Us

The symbolism of the lotus flower is extremely important in yoga. The lotus flower is a beautiful circle of petals that floats on a lake. The lotus's roots, however, are deep in the mud. This mud provides the nutrients to help the lotus grow and achieve its beauty. To *yogis*, the lotus represents human life. Our lives are submerged in "mud"—in the material world, in striving and grasping, in worry and pain. Yet we can use these challenges the way the lotus root absorbs nutrients from the mud—sending up a shoot that will ride to the top of the murky lake and bloom on the surface in perfect beauty.

Maybe inner joy isn't what you're looking for. Maybe you don't even believe it's something that's possible for you to find. Yoga doesn't turn you into anything you aren't. Yoga simply releases you so you can find the joy that everyone has inside. Yoga is a personal journey, and you go at your own pace. All you have to do is follow the map; that is, practice the postures. Meditate, if you feel like you're ready. Gradually, as you become prepared, the joy—the inner delight—will come.

The Least You Need to Know

➤ Yoga uses the fight-or-flight response to your benefit.

➤ Yoga teaches mindfulness.

➤ Meditation is simply relaxation for your mind.

➤ Meditation stimulates *vidya*—correct understanding—and dispels negative thoughts, feelings, and actions.

➤ Practicing yoga poses with your full attention can help you learn how to achieve flow, or total absorption and optimal skill in whatever you are doing.

Part 2

Let's Get Spiritual: Growing with the Tree of Yoga

This section begins with a mini history lesson. Yoga has been around for thousands of years, and in all that time, it has branched into various types, from studious Jnana Yoga *to active* Karma Yoga *to mystical* Kundalini Yoga. *Learn about how yoga came to the West and why our culture is coming to a point in its evolution where yoga will become a powerful and pertinent tool.*

Next we introduce you to yoga's comprehensive guidelines for living. Far from hard-and-fast "commandments," yoga's yamas *(abstinences) and* niyamas *(observances) point the way along the path that will most enhance your yoga journey. Patanjali's Eightfold Path (of which the abstinences and observances are the first two aspects) is laid out in an easy-to-follow format, explaining the eight important facets of a yogi's life—from keeping the body fit to mastering detachment, concentration, and meditation.*

Controlling the breath keeps body and mind operating at peak efficiency. In Chapter 7, "Can You Breathe?" we explain the how's and why's of the yoga system of breath control called pranayama. *Chapter 8, "Hatha Yoga:* May the Force Be with You," *goes on to describe the details of* Hatha Yoga, *a system of yoga emphasizing control of the body and the most popular form of yoga in the West.*

Chapter 5

Going Back in Time: The Yoga Tradition

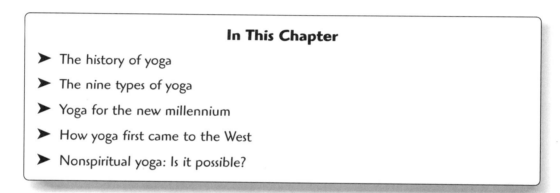

In This Chapter

➤ The history of yoga

➤ The nine types of yoga

➤ Yoga for the new millennium

➤ How yoga first came to the West

➤ Nonspiritual yoga: Is it possible?

You don't have to know anything about the yoga tradition to practice yoga. After all, we're not in school and we're not going to give you any kind of history test. But history can be interesting, especially when there *isn't* a test—no pressure! Yoga's history is particularly illustrious and ancient. Understanding the deep and sagacious roots of your fitness program may help you gain a deeper appreciation of yoga's staying power and sacred origins.

People Practiced Yoga in 2500 B.C.E.

Yoga has been around for a long, long time. "How long?" you ask. The *Rig-Veda* is quite possibly the oldest-known text in the world, and it contains definite elements of yoga. Although the only remaining written versions are a few hundred years old, the earliest hymns are believed to be over 4,000 years old. The hymns of the *Rig-Veda* were passed down via an oral tradition, with great accuracy. Hindu priests were trained to memorize the hymns to the letter. If the *Rig-Veda* is indeed thousands of years old, its existence may coincide with the existence of the Vedic people who lived along the Indus River and also with the *Pyramid Texts,* thought to be the oldest written documents in existence.

But just because yoga is old doesn't mean it's old-fashioned. Yoga is timeless, transcending cultures, eras, and philosophies. They say you never know if something will be a classic until it has stood the test of time. Need we say more?

Yoga Studies All Religions

Yoga may seem like a religion. It offers guidelines for living, spirituality, study of sacred texts, and communion with the "divine." Some branches of yoga seem more religious or mystical than others, but yoga itself isn't a religion.

Yoga is open to all religions and encourages the study of all religious and spiritual texts. Yoga is not biased, prejudiced, or exclusive. You needn't be a Hindu, a Muslim, a Christian, or a Jew, but you may be any of these. Whatever religion you practice, yoga will help you understand your beliefs more clearly and get you in closer touch with your spiritual side.

In Search of the Sacred (*Svadhyaya*)

Because yoga encourages the study of the sacred (*svadhyaya*), it may be helpful for you to become at least somewhat familiar with the major spiritual texts. Reading and studying any or all of them will benefit your yoga practice by expanding your mind to possibilities you may not have considered.

Know Your Sanskrit

Svadhyaya (pronounced *svahd-YAH-yah*) means "inquiring into your own nature, the nature of your beliefs, and the nature of the world's spiritual journey." Accomplished by the study of sacred texts, such as the *Bhagavad Gita* and the Bible, as well as through self-contemplation, *svadhyaya* is one of yoga's observances and one aspect of Patanjali's Eightfold Path, as described in the *Yoga Sutra* (and further explained in Chapter 6, "Walking Yoga's Eightfold Path").

We aren't saying you should give up your other pursuits and devote your life to the minute study of ancient religious scriptures (unless you think that sounds like fun). However, reading the sacred texts of our world, or even just those of your own religion, can help you get in touch with the spiritual journey our species has undergone since we were first able to comprehend the concepts of spirituality, divinity, and the universe.

Here are a few of the major sacred texts of India (since that's where yoga really blossomed, and many of these texts directly mention yoga or its concepts):

➤ The *Rig-Veda,* considered the most ancient of sacred texts. Meaning "Knowledge of Praise," it's been orally passed down via sages who memorized it. Consisting of 1,028 hymns, the *Rig-Veda* is now believed to be over 4,000 years old.

➤ The *Upanishads,* the scriptures of ancient Hindu philosophy, which describes the path of *Jnana Yoga,* the discipline of wisdom as a path to self-realization.

➤ The *Bhagavad Gita,* perhaps the most famous Hindu text and the epic story of *Arjuna,* a warrior-prince, who confronts moral dilemmas and is led to a better understanding of reality through the intercession of the god *Krishna.*

Wise Yogi Tells Us

The *Bhagavad Gita* is one of India's most beloved sacred texts. It tells the epic story of the warrior-prince *Arjuna* as he stands at the edge of a battlefield preparing for war. He discusses his universal moral dilemmas with the Hindu god, *Krishna,* who is driving *Arjuna's* chariot. Is war justified? What if your loved ones are on the opposing side? What is right when your duties conflict? What does it mean to be born, to live, to die? The *Bhagavad Gita* is widely available and still a good read. (And it isn't even very long!) Pick up a copy and see what the fuss is all about. It's a beautiful story of inner quests and spiritual awakenings.

➤ The *Yoga Sutra* of Patanjali, the source of Patanjali's Eightfold Path. Many call Patanjali the father of yoga because of this significant and influential text, but yoga was around long before Patanjali, who only made it more accessible.

➤ The *Hatha-Yoga-Pradipika,* a fourteenth-century guide to *Hatha Yoga*—everything you always wanted to know about *Hatha Yoga* but were afraid to ask!

Planting the Seeds: Yoga Branches for All Growing Personalities

Up to this point, although we've been focusing primarily on *Hatha Yoga*, we haven't really been distinguishing between all the different types of yoga. Yoga has a unified goal (a state of pure bliss and oneness with the universe), but each of the various methods emphasizes a different way to get to that goal.

Hatha Yoga: *Know Your Body, Know Your Mind*

As we've mentioned before, *Hatha Yoga* works under the assumption that supreme control over the body, or the physical self, is one path to enlightenment. *Hatha Yoga* is a sort of spiritual fitness plan in which balance is a key. Attention to the physical is foremost in *Hatha Yoga;* this particular type of yoga involves cleansing rituals and breathing exercises designed to manipulate the body's energy through breath control, in addition to the postures or exercises for which *Hatha Yoga* is commonly known.

Wise Yogi Tells Us

If you're ill, whether you have a cold, chronic pain, or something more serious, *Hatha Yoga* postures, meditation, and the practice of mindfulness can be of great benefit. Learning to relax, physically and mentally, can comfort you and aid in healing. If you're in physical pain due to illness, however, or find yourself too distracted to even think about meditating, start slow, as little as five minutes a day. Even taking a series of full, deep breaths can be centering to body and mind.

Raja Yoga: *Know Your Mind, Know the Universe*

Raja Yoga, also known as *The Royal Path,* emphasizes control of the intellect to attain enlightenment. Meditation, concentration, and breath control are paramount in *Raja Yoga,* the yoga of the mind. *Hatha* and *Raja Yoga* work well together; *Hatha Yoga* is often considered a stepping stone to *Raja Yoga,* because after control of the body is mastered, control of the mind comes more easily.

Kriya Yoga *and* Karma Yoga: *Act It Out!*

Kriya Yoga and *Karma Yoga* are the yogas of action. *Kriya* means "spiritual action," and *Kriya Yoga* involves the practice of quieting the mind through scriptural self-study, breathing techniques, *mantras,* and meditation. *Kriya Yoga* understands that divine energy is stored in the lower part of the body. The study of *Kriya Yoga* breathing and meditation techniques helps to bring this energy up the spine. As the energy builds, the *yogi's* body (physical and astral) is strengthened.

In *Karma Yoga,* the emphasis is selfless action. *Karma Yoga* transcends concerns of success or failure, egoism, and selfishness. What emerges is service to all beings. Because yoga teaches that every person is part of the divine universal spirit, *Karma Yoga* encourages that all beings on this earth be served with the respect deserving of a divine presence. The follower of *Karma Yoga* proceeds through daily life attempting to increase virtue and decrease lawlessness in the world by working for others and foregoing personal desires, resulting in greater empathy for and understanding of the world—and eventually, full understanding, or enlightenment.

Know Your Sanskrit

Karma is the law of cause and effect, or "what goes around comes around." Everything you do, say, or think has an immediate effect in the universe and in you. *Karma* is not negative. It is neither bad nor good. It is the movement toward balanced consciousness.

Bhakti Yoga: *Open Your Heart*

Bhakti Yoga places sincere, heartfelt devotion to the divine ahead of all else. *Bhakti Yoga* involves reverence, devotion, and perpetual remembrance of whatever divine presence is meaningful to you. Unsettled minds, intellectual concerns, the material world—all fall away as love takes over and the heart is enveloped in thoughts of the divine. The heart is *Bhakti Yoga*'s focus and is cultivated as the primary way to achieve unity with the divine.

Jnana Yoga: *Sagacious You*

Jnana Yoga is the path of knowledge and wisdom. Inquiring minds are what *Jnana Yoga* is all about, and because all knowledge is hidden within us, *Jnana Yoga*'s goal is to inquire deeply into ourselves through questioning, meditation, and contemplation until we find that knowledge. *Jnana Yoga* involves a radical shift in perception. Everything you know, think, believe, or feel is questioned—temporarily. When everything you know is suddenly untrue, all that remains is you and the universe, which are the same thing. The goal is wisdom, which is far beyond the mere accumulation of information. It's direct knowledge of the divine through the elimination of all that is merely illusion.

Tantra, Mantra, *and* Kundalini Yoga

Tantra, Mantra, and *Kundalini Yoga* are grouped together here because they are all somewhat different than the other types of yoga. Although they share many practices and ideas, *Tantra, Mantra,* and *Kundalini Yoga* are more esoteric than other forms of yoga. *Tantra Yoga* involves the study of sacred writings and rituals. *Mantra Yoga* is the study of sacred sounds. *Kundalini Yoga* is the study of *kundalini* (energy) movement

53

along the spine, which is released through breath and specific *Hatha Yoga* movements. All three types of yoga should be learned under the guidance of a qualified teacher and all require a degree of emotional, mental, and moral preparation.

Tantra Yoga has been associated with sexual rituals in popular culture, but that is an inaccurate portrayal. *Tantric* thought assumes that we live in a dark age (*kali yuga*) and therefore must use every method possible to boost our spirituality. Because *Tantra Yoga* emphasizes the power of ritual, it has become most famous in Western culture for its notion that sexual energy is an important store of energy that can be rechanneled to further you along your way to spiritual enlightenment. Our culture has expanded on the idea of sexual energy and sometimes perverts the concept into something it was never meant to be. *Tantra* isn't about sex. It is a complex, ancient, and esoteric discipline with a wide range of practices, often involving sacred rituals based on the idea that humans are reflections of divinity.

Tantra is also meant to be studied under a qualified adept, and its rituals and philosophies kept secret from others who aren't receiving professional guidance; the intention is to prevent its precepts from being misunderstood and misused.

Know Your Sanskrit

Tantra means "technique," and **Tantra Yoga** involves the techniques of ritual and study to eliminate obstacles to enlightenment. **Kali yuga** (pronounced *KAH-lee YOO-gah*) is the fourth of four ages (*yuga* means "age") and the age in which we are now living. The shortest of all the ages, *kali yuga* is 432,000 years long. The other ages are **satya yuga,** the first age (1,728,000 years); **treta yuga,** the second age (1,296,000 years); and **dvapara yuga,** the third age (864,000 years).

Mantra Yoga centers around the principle that sound can affect consciousness. *Shamanism,* yoga's probable precursor, considered sound an extremely important aspect of the search for spiritual enlightenment, and even today many religions use singing, chanting, rhythm, and recitation in their rituals. *Mantra Yoga* arose as a result of mystical experiences rather than philosophy. A *mantra* is a syllable or sequence of syllables designed to clear the mind and encourage spiritual awakening. Sanskrit syllables are thought to awaken reflexology points in the mouth, which in turn energize the body to higher states of consciousness. *Om* is the most commonly known *mantra* syllable and sounds curiously (but probably not coincidentally) like "Amen," the sound that punctuates so many religious hymns and prayers.

Om, written in Sanskrit.

Chanting a *mantra* puts you in touch with the vibrational patterns of the world and the universe's ocean of vibration, helping you ascend to a state of oneness with the universe. *Mantra Yoga* is all about that vibration and the sonic aspect of the divine.

Japa is the process of repeating *mantras* over and over for the purpose of clearing the mind. Here are a few *mantras* other than *Om* that you might like to try:

Know Your Sanskrit

Shamanism (pronounced *SHAH–mahn–ihzm*) is the religion of certain northeast Asian peoples, based on the philosophy that the workings of good and evil spirits can be influenced, but only by *shamans* (*SHAH–mahns*), the priests of shamanism.

➤ OM NAMAH SHIVAYA (pronounced *OHM NAH-mah SHEE-vah-YAH*). "To divinity my salutations again and again."

➤ HARI-OM (*HAH-ree OHM*). "Preserving goodness in all."

➤ OM NAMO BHAGAVATE VASUDEVAYA (*OHM NAH-moh BAH-GAH-VAH-teh VAH-soo-DEE-VAH-yah*). "I turn to the divinity within the heart of all beings."

➤ AHAM BRAHMASMI (*AH-HAM BRAH-MAHS-mee*). "I am the absolute."

➤ OM MANI PADME HUM (*OHM MAH-nee PAHD-may HOOM*). "Enlightened body, enlightened speech, enlightened mind, active compassion."

Kundalini Yoga involves techniques meant to awaken the energy, symbolized as a snake, that "sleeps" at the base of the spine. When released correctly (that is, when the recipient is properly prepared), *kundalini* energy, sometimes called "serpent power," is potent and results in enlightenment. If released too soon, *kundalini* energy mixes with a person's negative emotionality and can turn into intense and painful experiences.

Pure *kundalini* is a balanced and compassionate state of being. A person cannot have a negative *kundalini* experience. If someone has a negative experience, it is due to something other than *kundalini*. A *kundalini* awakening is thought to result not only in enlightenment, but also in the ability to control involuntary bodily functions such as heartbeat.

Know Your Sanskrit

Kundalini is energy that lies curled like a snake at the base of the spine and can be awakened through various techniques and movements, after which it travels up the spine, activating the *chakras*. *Kundalini Yoga* is specifically designed to release this energy and channel it.

To awaken the *kundalini,* you must go through complex mental and breathing exercises that should be practiced only under the guidance of a qualified teacher. Sometimes (though it's rare), a *kundalini* awakening will happen spontaneously, but don't be scared away. *Kundalini Yoga* is, at its heart, searching for the same thing as all other types of yoga. Classes are available in this interesting branch of yoga; with proper instruction, the practice of *Kundalini Yoga* can be enjoyable, energizing, and ultimately enlightening.

Why Practicing Yoga Is So Twenty-First Century

We would describe the twenty-first–century world as materialistic but optimistic. As people gradually become disillusioned by, or recover from, materialism, discovering that it doesn't bring happiness, they are searching, in increasing numbers, for a way of life more satisfying and fulfilling. So you've got the Porsche, the penthouse, the beachfront condo, and the three-carat diamond. Now what? Or maybe you've gone through a bankruptcy or divorce, and you're starting over. Stuff didn't make you happy. Relationships based on stuff, illusions, and nonreality didn't work, either. Now what?

Throughout history, priorities change and fashions come and go. The pendulum is swinging back toward spiritual priorities and self-actualization, away from more worldly concerns. This trend is apparent in the popularity of books like this one, on subjects both spiritual and holistic. People are looking inward again.

Yoga fits easily and comfortably into these new (or renewed) priorities. Yoga doesn't (or shouldn't) concern itself with technology, wealth, or sophistication. It's an inner journey toward self-realization and an outer journey toward physical control, holistic health, and confidence that comes not from possessions but from self-possession.

East Meets West

Nineteenth-century America was largely unfamiliar with Eastern thought. Then, in 1893, *Swami* Vivekananda addressed the Parliament of Religions, causing quite a sensation. He quickly became a popular figure and was followed by a number of other *swamis* who came to the United States to teach and guide Westerners along the Eastern path of yoga. *Swami* Vivekananda was followed by many other *gurus* who came to the West and profoundly influenced their followers, such as *Swami* Paramahansa Yogananda, *Swami* Sivananda, and many more.

The 1960s rock group The Beatles became interested in Eastern thought and even visited India, befriending *Maharishi* Mahesh Yogi. George Harrison in particular was fascinated with Indian culture. He became enamored with the *sitar* (a Hindu stringed instrument that looks a little bit like a mandolin), and was one of the first to bring *sitar* music into rock and roll. The Beatles, through songs such as "Norwegian Wood (This Bird Has Flown)" and "Within You, Without You," introduced Hindu melodies to modern music and opened Westerners' minds to different sounds and new experiences.

The *Maharishi* came to the West in 1959. America's "hippie generation" took to yoga in the 1960s, perhaps because traditional values were being questioned and yoga offered an alternative set of values attractive to spiritual seekers. After a few decades of excessive materialism and a world of violence, drug abuse, broken families, and the notable absence of any firmly held spiritual beliefs, yoga is more popular than ever before. We are seeking the spiritual with new vigor as an answer to a world we can't control.

Can You Do Yoga Without Being Spiritual?

"All right, all right," you may be saying, "I'm interested in yoga, but this whole spiritual angle just isn't *me*." Worry not. You can do yoga without being spiritual, even though yoga is traditionally a spiritual pursuit. The postures, as we've said before, are great for fitness. Breathing exercises have wonderful physiological benefits. Even meditation needn't be spiritual—just a fitness program for the mind.

Know Your Sanskrit

Swami is correctly spelled "svamin," but Westerners say *swami*. *Svamin* is a title of respect for a spiritual person who is master of himself rather than of others. **Guru** literally means "dispeller of darkness." *Gurus* are self-realized adepts who initiate others into self-realization.

Wise Yogi Tells Us

Maharishi Mahesh Yogi was the inventor of Transcendental Meditation, or TM, which involves the mental repetition of a *mantra*. A *mantra* can be provided to you by your TM instructor, or you can create your own. TM is a great way to achieve deep relaxation, and TM instructors are widely available to teach you the technique.

Yoga is so personal that it's impossible to say what it "should" be for anyone. In fact, yoga is distinctly "anti-should." It involves doing what feels right for you, what you want to do. The purpose of yoga is to maximize your potential—to help the best possible *you* emerge. Maybe the best possible you has no use for spiritual enlightenment. Whatever your potential, whatever your gifts, yoga will help you find them and make the most of them.

The Least You Need to Know

➤ Yoga is really, really old but still really, really relevant.

➤ Different types of yoga—*Hatha, Raja, Kriya, Karma, Bhakti, Jnana, Tantra, Mantra,* and *Kundalini*—emphasize different practices but have the same goal: enlightenment.

➤ You don't have to be spiritual to practice yoga, but if you practice yoga, you'll probably end up being a little more spiritual.

Chapter 6

Walking Yoga's Eightfold Path

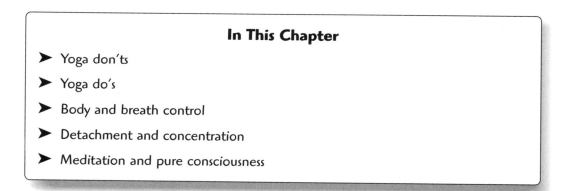

In This Chapter

➤ Yoga don'ts

➤ Yoga do's

➤ Body and breath control

➤ Detachment and concentration

➤ Meditation and pure consciousness

If you're the kind of person who likes a nice, clean set of rules to live by, this is the chapter for you! In Patanjali's *Yoga Sutra,* the eight limbs of yoga are enumerated. These limbs provide a structure for your yoga practice and your daily life. They are designed to help you along the yoga path. One very important thing to remember about the eight limbs of yoga: They are *not* commandments or laws! They are more like guidelines for living. But if you don't follow the guidelines, it doesn't constitute any sort of "sin." The Yoga Police won't come to your house and arrest you. Success with your yoga practice will simply be easier if you live your life according to Patanjali's suggestions.

However, if you don't want to meditate, give up meat, or even relinquish your materialistic nature, don't pressure yourself. Remember that yoga is not only a practice, but something that happens to you. As you progress and grow, you may find that you're naturally less materialistic, you lose interest in eating meat, or you become drawn to meditation as the next logical step in your journey. Maybe those things won't happen. Maybe for now, you just want to tackle the suggestions one at a time. No hurry!

And for those of you who want some commandments and want them *now*, it's also fine to view Patanjali's Eightfold Path more stringently. It all depends on who you are and what kind of thinking you're most likely to respond to.

Yoga Don'ts: Just Say No (Yamas)

First we'll talk about Patanjali's suggested abstinences. This is a difficult category for a lot of people who want to do yoga but don't want to be bound to any restrictions. Again, the abstinences, or *yamas*, aren't rules meant to limit you. They are suggestions meant to help you grow by purifying your body and mind. Practicing them can teach you self-discipline. You may also find that you already live by many of them.

Do No Harm (Ahimsa)

The first *yama* is about nonviolence. "That's an easy one," you say? Well, nonviolence means more than keeping yourself from beating up your obnoxious neighbor when he won't turn down his stereo. We can be violent in many ways, often without realizing it.

Ahimsa involves nonviolent actions, nonviolent words, and nonviolent thoughts. Nonviolent actions involve the obvious—don't physically hurt people. (Not even when they hurt you first.) Nonviolence isn't exactly about turning the other cheek. It's more like dodging the punch. For some, nonviolent action also means vegetarianism, because meat was once an animal, bird, or fish that was killed. Killing is violence. But if this step is too big for you, don't worry about it for now. Concentrate on eliminating violence in other ways. You'll come to understand the full range of opportunities for nonviolence at your own pace.

Nonviolent words are also important. Nonviolent speech means refraining from words that slander, degrade, or hurt another person. A good rule of thumb is to "honey-coat" your words, because you may have to eat them later! But that doesn't mean lying. You needn't tell your Aunt Maude that her polyester pantsuit is the most lovely outfit you've ever seen—she may give you one for your next birthday! And what if she asks you what you think about it? "Aunt Maude, that outfit is definitely *you!*"

Nonviolent thoughts are equally important. Aunt Maude can't hear you thinking, "If I had taste like that, I would never leave my house!" The trouble with your thoughts, though, is that they pervade your entire being and are notoriously difficult to control. Having nonviolent thoughts means refusing to wish harm to anyone, even if you really think they deserve it. (Oops! That's bordering on a violent thought right there!) Let your negative thoughts go, wish your enemies well (even in the privacy of your own brain), and your heart will lighten. According to yoga, we are energy, and our thoughts can be sensed on an energetic level, so they are impossible to hide completely. People sense what you're thinking, so you're better off transforming your negative thoughts than trying to hide them. The beautiful thing about yoga is that your awareness becomes heightened and you perceive the thoughts of others more clearly, too (of course, that could reveal some things you'd rather not know, but in the service of truth, we say it's worth it).

And one more thing about nonviolence: Engaging in negative talk and thoughts about yourself ("I am ugly," "I am lazy," "I can't do anything right") is doing violence to yourself. It counts—don't do it!

A Yoga Minute

Scientific studies have shown that large groups practicing organized meditation in one location reduce social stress and violence.

Tell No Lies (Satya)

The second *yama* involves truthfulness. But what is the truth? You and I have different truths, so isn't truth changeable? According to yoga philosophy, truthfulness is the result of our mind, speech, and actions being unified and harmonious. According to yoga philosophy, truth does no harm. This results in personal integrity and strength of character.

Check out these scenarios and see if any of them are familiar:

➤ Someone confides in you and you promise you won't tell his or her secret, but then you don't "count" your spouse or your best friend. You've said the words, "I'm not supposed to tell you this, but ...."

➤ You receive an extra $10 bill with your grocery change or at the bank and walk quickly away. After all, you need the $10 more than that big corporation!

➤ You occasionally bend or creatively interpret the rules on your income taxes just a little.

➤ You tell poor Aunt Maude you aren't feeling well and can't possibly visit her this week, even though you're actually feeling just fine.

Most of us have had at least occasional instances when it seemed more convenient, easier, or even kinder to bend the truth (or just snap it right in two!). It isn't easy to suddenly wake up one morning, vow to act completely truthfully, and then stick to your vow. You can start by becoming more aware of what you're doing. Ask yourself, "Is this harmonious with all parts of me? Does this do no harm?" If you aren't sure, maybe you should hold back. Dig deeper for the real truth in your daily life.

Just like everyone around you, you are so much more complex than your outward appearance, your job, the face you show the world, or the opinions others have of you. What seems to be the truth—what is obviously the truth, what you know is the truth—often is not the truth at all. Truth is tricky, but it's out there, buried under layers of misrepresentations, grudges, low self-esteem, unfortunate experiences, negative input, and discomforts. Striving for truth and bliss in your everyday life will help those layers fall away. Living truthfully takes some effort, but you can do it!

There are absolute truths that one perceives in the stillness of one's being. We're all searching for truth, and it's within everyone's grasp.

No More Stealing (Asteya)

So you think you don't steal? Just because you've never shoplifted a candy bar or a car radio doesn't mean you don't steal. The concept is simple, even if the implications aren't: If it's not yours, don't take it. (We assume we needn't mention that this *yama* includes no robbing banks or holding up armored cars!) That means no shoplifting, and no taking credit for someone else's creations or ideas (plagiarizing), or for anything else anyone has done or said. Don't interrupt people and steal their center of attention. Don't steal your child's chance to do something on his own by doing it for him. Your actions affect this world—don't forget that.

Cool It, Casanova (Brahmacharya)

Brahmacharya is about chastity. No, don't close the book and toss it aside! This *yama* doesn't mean telling your spouse the fun is over and you now need separate beds. *Brahmacharya* is about virtue, and not just when it comes to sex. Many great *yogis* are householders, which means they are married … with children.

Brahma means "truth," and *car* means "to move," so *brahmacharya* essentially means "to control the movement of truth." Lust and desire, in their many forms, obscure truth. Developing the inner strength to control our lusts and desires helps us to see truth more clearly. In other words, *brahmacharya* is a movement toward responsible behavior and a higher truth beyond the physical, the force of "I want" in life. The *Bhagavad Gita* describes this *yama* in the following way:

> "While contemplating the objects of the senses, a person develops attachment for them, and from such attachment, lust develops, and from lust, anger arises. From anger, delusion arises, and from delusion, bewilderment of memory. When memory is bewildered, intelligence is lost, and when intelligence is lost, one falls down again into the material pool."

Being virtuous means holding the opposite sex in high esteem and nurturing respect for someone you love. It also means holding *yourself* in high esteem and refusing to let your body be swayed by its every whim, desire, and want, whether that desire is for a person or for power or for a pound of Hershey's Kisses. Refusing to let your body be swayed by desire certainly doesn't preclude sex, a good promotion, or chocolate, for that matter. Instead, this *yama* encourages the kind of restraint and attitude towards those things we tend to desire that will help keep our minds clear and focused.

The *brahmacharya yama* is often described as being about sex, and technically, it does preclude sexual lust—the one-night stand, using people sexually (including yourself), and all the other things we typically associate with the word "lust." Letting your desire for sex consume you is no way to become self-aware or calm and centered! But *brahmacharya* also encompasses lusts and desires of all kinds. At the very heart of this *yama*, desire itself, no matter its object, is what keeps us from seeing truth. To master our desires is to gain self-awareness.

Ouch!

Engaging in meaningless physical contact may only lead you away from the possibility of encountering someone who could become a life partner.

Don't Be Greedy (Aparigraha)

Go to your closet and count the pairs of shoes lined up in there—or the red sweaters or white shirts or ties. Or maybe you can't even open the closet because it's bursting with *stuff*. It isn't easy to abstain from greed in this materialistic world. With television, radio, and billboards continually telling us what we want and what we must have, it's hard not to believe some of it. But are you familiar with the feeling of buying something you've always wanted, then feeling strangely dissatisfied, as if the fun was in the wanting, not in the actual possessing? That is greed's payoff—emptiness.

Nongreed means living simply, possessing only what is necessary, and recognizing that possessions are merely tools to use in life. Accumulations, whether material things or unnecessary thoughts, tie you down to this world. Simplify your life as you simplify your thoughts.

Know Your Sanskrit

Yamas (pronounced YAH-mahs) are five abstinences or forms of discipline that purify the body and mind: **ahimsa** (ah-HIM-sah) means "nonviolence," **satya** (SAHT-ya) means "truthfulness," **asteya** (ah-STAY-yah) means "nonstealing," **brahmacharya** (BRAH-mah-CHAR-yah) means "chastity or nonlust," and **aparigraha** (ah-PAH-ree-GRAH-hah) means "nongreed."

Greed can also surface in less obvious ways. Talking too much, interrupting others, and dominating conversations while barely showing a flicker of interest in the participation of others are all ways greed creeps into our lives through language. Think before you speak, and consider how your words will sound and what effect they will have. Practice listening and being truly present in a conversation, absorbing everything other people are saying.

Thoughts can also be a source of greed. How come the Smiths have a swimming pool and a fancy two-level deck, while you have to sit on the back stoop under the sprinkler? Why did your best friend get diamonds for her birthday when you only got a toaster? Envy and jealousy clutter the mind and can become obsessions. How much better it is to turn those feelings around and feel truly happy for the person who has something you don't have! In fact, once you start to be happy for someone else simply because of their joy, you may become so fulfilled by your happiness that you lose your desire for whatever they have. How much simpler your life becomes when you can be happy due to something beyond your own needs!

Yoga Do's: Just Say Yes (Niyamas)

And now for the fun part! *Niyamas* are Patanjali's observances—what to do, as opposed to what *not* to do. The first *niyama* cleanses the way for all the others.

Be Pure (Shauca)

Purity is achieved through the practice of the five previous *yamas,* so the *yamas* and *niyamas* work hand in hand. The abstentions clear away negative physical and mental states of being, leading you straight to purity. Purity can apply to various aspects of your life. Cleanliness is very important to yoga. Keeping yourself clean by bathing; dressing in fresh, clean clothes; and keeping your surroundings clean are all part of pure actions.

What you eat is also important. Fresh, natural, and healthy foods are best. Foods obtained through nonviolent means are ideal because they can be eaten with full, unadulterated joy; this is why *yogis* traditionally practice a vegetarian diet. Of course, if you want to get "yoga-technical," vegetables are alive, too (all life is to be respected, revered, and appreciated, and all life is interconnected), so respect each meal for the life given to sustain another.

Be Content (Santosha)

Just saying the word *santosha* invokes a feeling of calm. Practicing contentment means finding happiness with what you have and with who you are. Of course, you can always work toward improvement, but that doesn't mean you can't be content while you're improving yourself! Contentment helps you see that you're exactly where you're supposed to be right now. It doesn't mean you'll be happy when you can finally stand on your head, get that promotion, or find a soulmate. It means happiness in this moment, as you are.

Contentment means learning to reevaluate obstacles as opportunities. Limitations are learning experiences. Easier said than done, we know! If you feel unhappy with your life, you may find it especially difficult to cultivate contented thoughts. Practicing contentment involves taking full responsibility for your life and the situations you're in. Find the positives in life's lessons and choose to grow from them. You're in charge of your own destiny, but that also means not beating yourself up for the "mess" you're in. Thank yourself for it. Laugh! Know that every situation or challenge presented is a doorway to greater growth.

Wise Yogi Tells Us

Feeling discontented? Try this exercise. Create a list of everything that makes you discontented. Then rewrite your list, finding a way to see each source of discontentment in some positive light. For example, rewrite "I hate my job" to say "My job has taught me I am more creative than I thought." When you're finished, throw away that first list—you don't need it!

Be Disciplined (Tapas)

For all the *yamas* and *niyamas* to be truly effective, you'll need a little self-discipline. Not your strong point? If self-discipline were easy, what would be the point? It would hardly be discipline.

Anyone who exercises daily is showing self-discipline. Dedicating a specific time each day to your yoga practice is self-discipline. But how many times have you started an exercise program, only to abandon it as soon as it got boring or tedious? Learning how to stick to something even when you don't feel like it will build your strength and wisdom. You probably manage the self-discipline to brush your teeth twice every day. Just extend that discipline, bit by bit, to other aspects of your life, one step at a time. Maybe tomorrow you'll brush your teeth and have a healthy salad for lunch. Maybe next week you'll be brushing your teeth, eating salads, and doing 10 minutes of yoga. By next year, there's no telling what you can accomplish.

Disciplined words mean speaking gently and sincerely, not angrily or hurtfully. *Act* rather than *react,* because you cannot control the actions of others. Self-disciplined thoughts replace the negative with the positive, resentment with forgiveness, violence with peace, and unhappiness with joy.

The *yamas* and *niyamas* themselves provide an excellent opportunity to practice self-discipline.

Wise Yogi Tells Us

Self-discipline is difficult for almost everyone, but changing your attitude may help keep you on track. The best way to do this is to focus on the positive: "I will spend 30 minutes practicing yoga today." "I will relax with deep-breathing exercises tonight before I go to bed." "I will have a soothing cup of herbal tea this morning." Focusing on the positive makes being disciplined more fun. Because really, discipline isn't deprivation, it's self-care.

Be Studious (Svadhyaya)

Svadhyaya doesn't just mean you should read a lot of books. It means studying yourself through introspection. Do you act according to your beliefs? Do you say what you mean? Are you walking your talk? Studious action means paying attention to your physical self. How are you sitting, standing, or walking? Do you feel graceful or stilted? Do you look the way you feel? If not, why not? Studious words and thoughts involve the study of various sacred texts—whichever are relevant to you— to inspire and teach you. Through self-study, you can see which thoughts, actions, words, and experiences actually make you happy, and which block your happiness. Dedicated, nonviolent introspection will fill your life with clarity.

Know Your Sanskrit

Niyamas are observances or personal disciplines. Again, there are five: **shauca** (pronounced SAH-chah) means "purity, or inner and outer cleanliness"; **santosha** (san-TOH-shah) means "contentment"; **tapas** (TAH-pahs) means "self-discipline"; **svadhyaya** (svahd-YAH-yah) means "self-study"; and **ishvara-pranidhana** (ISH-var-ah PRAH-nee-DAH-nah) means "centering on the divine."

Be Devoted (Ishvara-Pranidhana)

The last *niyama* involves devotion. Focus on the divine, whatever that means to you—how it is in you and part of you and all around you. *Ishvara-pranidhana* is an observance that works beautifully with any religion. Whether you're devoted to God, Buddha, or the Force, this *niyama* reminds you to relinquish ego and center on your highest ideal. Positive energy will flow from the divine into all areas of your life.

Eightfold Path At-a-Glance

1. Yoga Don'ts (*Yamas*)
   No violence
   No lying
   No stealing
   No pursuit of lust/desire
   No greed
2. Yoga Do's (*Niyamas*)
   Purity
   Contentment
   Self-Discipline
   Self-Study
   Devotion
3. Yoga Poses (*Asanas*)
4. Breathing Exercises (*Pranayama*)
5. Detachment (*Pratyahara*)
6. Concentration (*Dharana*)
7. Meditation (*Dhyana*)
8. Pure Consciousness (*Samadhi*)

Are You Wearing Your Walking Shoes? More Yoga Pathways

But what about the rest of the Eightfold Path? Technically, so far we've covered only the first two limbs. The remaining limbs of the Eightfold Path are also important and complete the framework for the modern practice of yoga.

Growing with yoga's Eightfold Path.

Body Control (Asanas)

We've already talked about body control, or the *asanas,* as both an important part of yoga and its most well-known component. Remember that body control is not the only path, but merely one path yoga offers. Yet body control is very important and makes a great starting point for any aspiring *yogi. Asana* literally translates as "posture" and is derived from the Sanskrit root *as,* which means "to stay." Patanjali describes an *asana* as having *sthira* and *sukha,* or steadiness and the ability to remain comfortable. Remember these two qualities when practicing your postures, keeping in mind the very important *yama* of *ahimsa,* or nonviolence: Never work to the point of pain, because that is doing violence to your body.

Breath Control (Pranayama)

Pranayama is another important path. *Prana* refers to the life force or energy that exists everywhere and is manifested in each of us through the breath. *Ayama* means "to stretch or extend." *Prana* flows out from the body, and *pranayama* teaches us to maneuver and direct *prana* for optimal physical and mental benefit. After all, breathing is life. You can go for months without food, days without water, but only moments without breath. Breathing affects all our actions and our thoughts, too. Mastering your breath is an important step toward mastering the rest of yourself!

Ouch!

Are you feeling listless, depressed, and under the weather? According to ancient yoga texts, you have too much *prana* outside your body. *Prana* is constantly moving and flowing into and out of us, and *pranayama* is a tool for maintaining your health and well-being. Keep yourself healthier and happier by keeping more *prana* inside (where it belongs)!

Detachment (Pratyahara)

The fifth limb of yoga is sense-related. *Pratyahara* is the practice of withdrawing the senses from everything that stimulates them. Normally, we live by our senses. We are drawn to look at beautiful or even ugly things. We listen, we taste, we touch, and we smell. This is the ordinary state of things, but it's also a state we can temporarily suspend in favor of a deeper awareness. *Pratyahara* cuts off the connection between the senses and the brain. This can happen during breathing exercises, meditation, the practice of yoga postures, or any activity requiring concentration.

But what is the purpose of detaching ourselves from our senses? Aren't the senses good? They help us appreciate beauty, as when we watch a sunset, or warn us of danger, as when we smell smoke or spoiled food, and they permit us to communicate with each other. Unfortunately, our senses can also become so pleasurable that they control us instead of us controlling them. Maybe you enjoy your sensation of taste so much that you have become a little too obsessed with food. Maybe you love to talk but often talk so much that you forget to listen. Maybe you're addicted to television, caffeine, or sex.

Wise Yogi Tells Us

If the *yamas* and *niyamas* seem like a lot to remember, make yourself an abbreviated version of them—as plain or fancy as you like (framed calligraphy? computer graphics?)—and hang it up in your bedroom, bathroom, or wherever you'll see it each day. Or make a copy of the "Eightfold Path in Brief" chart in this chapter. Soon you'll have them memorized and they'll become a part of you.

Pratyahara wipes the sensual slate clean.

Detachment is also a great technique for pain control and an excellent way to deal with uncomfortable symptoms or chronic conditions. Try this technique for attaining sense withdrawal:

1. Sit erect. Place your thumbs on your ears, closing them off. Your eyes should be closed. Place your index fingers near your eyelashes to hold them gently shut and prevent movement of your eyeballs. (This assists the eyes in staying focused on the sun *chakra* or third eye. See Chapter 20, "*Chakras, Mudras, Mantras,* and *Mandalas.*") Each middle finger rests on the nasal passages. Your ring fingers are set on your upper lip and your little fingers on your lower lip.

2. Take a deep breath and gently press all fingers so your sense organs are suppressed. Turn inward, tuning out the external world. Focus your attention on your sun *chakra*.

3. When you can no longer comfortably hold your breath, release your fingers.

4. Exhale slowly. Inhale slowly. Repeat this gentle pressure for deeper reflections.

Concentration (Dharana)

Dhri means "to hold," and *dharana*, yoga's sixth limb, is all about learning to concentrate. Concentration involves teaching the mind to focus on one thing instead of many, as is our usual state of mind. *Dharana* is an exercise that can help with meditation. The goal is to become aware of nothing but the object on which you are concentrating, whether it's a candle flame, a flower, or a *mantra* you repeat to yourself.

The purpose is to train the mind to ignore all the extra, unnecessary junk floating around, to learn to gently push away superfluous thought. *Pratyahara* (withdrawal of the senses) is often the result when *dharana* is achieved, and both assist with more productive meditation, or *dhyana*.

Meditation (Dhyana)

Concentration is the exercise that leads to the state of meditation, and meditation techniques are, in essence, purity techniques. Meditation occurs when you've actually become linked to the object of your concentration so that nothing else exists. It's keen, heightened awareness, not nothingness. Your mind is completely focused and quiet but awake and aware of truth. Many methods exist to bring you to this state, but oneness with the object of your meditation, and subsequently, oneness with the entire universe, is the objective. And don't forget the wonderful fringe benefit of a calm and uncluttered mind able to think more quickly and see more clearly in all daily activities!

Know Your Sanskrit

Sthira (pronounced *STHIH-ra*) means "steadiness and alertness." **Sukha** (*SOO-kah*) means "lightness and comfort." Both are desirable qualities in yoga postures. **Pratyahara** (*PRAH-tyah-HAH-rah*) means "withdrawal of the senses"; **dharana** (*dah-RAH-nah*) means "orienting the mind toward a single point"; **dhyana** (*dee-YAH-nah*) means "meditation"; and **samadhi** (*sah-MAH-dee*) means "becoming one with the object of your meditation."

Pure Consciousness (Samadhi)

All the limbs of yoga lead to *samadhi*, the final limb of the Eightfold Path. *Samadhi* means "to merge," and this state of pure consciousness means just that: a complete and total merging with the object of your meditation.

When in a state of *samadhi*, you understand not only that you and the object of your meditation are one, but that you and the universe are one. There's no difference between you and everything else. How does this feel? Like a loss of identity? Yes, identity is meaningless in *samadhi*, but you won't be sorry. Who needs an ego when you have *samadhi*? *Samadhi* is pure, total bliss.

The Least You Need to Know

➤ Yoga offers guidelines for living.

➤ The five abstentions are nonviolence, not lying, not stealing, not lusting, and not being greedy.

➤ The five observances are purity, contentment, self-discipline, self-study, and devotion.

➤ Yoga also involves body control, breath control, detachment, concentration, and meditation.

➤ The goal of yoga is a deep, blissful oneness with the universe, which leads to liberation and self-realization.

Step 1:
INHALE.

Step 2:
EXHALE.

Can You Breathe?

Chapter 7

In This Chapter

➤ The universal energy of *prana*

➤ How *prana* makes you feel better

➤ Using *pranayama* to control *prana* in the body

➤ How to sit for optimal *pranayama*

➤ Some great *pranayama* techniques

Of course you can breathe ... or can you? Maybe well enough to get by without collapsing, but are you using your breath optimally? Probably not. Most people don't breathe as fully or deeply as they could, because it takes practice and concentration. Once you've learned the fine art of breath control, however, you'll certainly feel the difference.

An integral part of *Hatha Yoga* and other forms of yoga is *pranayama*, or breath control. In fact, the manipulation of breath to control the physical manifestation of *prana* in the body is *Hatha Yoga*'s realm. People in all cultures have learned to manipulate *prana*, either consciously or unconsciously. Faith healers, hypnotists, prophets, shamans, and spiritualists may use *prana*, although they may use another name for it. *Yogis* learn to use *prana* purposefully to push the mind to a higher state of consciousness. Speech can be charged with *prana*, which is why some people captivate us when they talk.

Prana, the Universal Life Force

In Chapter 6, "Walking Yoga's Eightfold Path," we described *prana* as the life force or energy that exists everywhere and is manifested in each of us through the breath, but *prana* isn't exactly the same thing as breath or oxygen. *Prana* exists in all living things. It doesn't have consciousness—it's pure energy. Every cell in your body is controlled by *prana*. *Prana* animates all matter. *Prana* can be a difficult concept to comprehend; it may become clearer if you understand what it isn't.

Once a body completely dies, administering oxygen won't bring it back to life, so obviously, oxygen doesn't equal life. Life is animated by more than oxygen—it's animated by *prana*. *Prana* is also not the matter it animates, nor the spirit it propels. *Prana* is universal energy that's in the air, in all matter, and is used by the spirit. You breathe in *prana* along with air, and *prana* regulates your body, from your nervous foot tapping the floor to your thoughts about your weekend plans.

We're now going to turn a little bit of attention to biology—biology according to yoga, that is. But don't get scared off; the concepts are easy to follow. Trust us.

Prana moves through the body along two energy pathways on either side of the spine. *Pingala* is on the right side and represents the sun. *Ida* is on the left side and represents the moon. In the middle is a passageway called *sushumna,* which runs through the spinal cord. Just picture a subway. The energy that keeps it running smoothly is *ida* and *pingala*. The *kundalini* is the train sitting at the bottom of this subway waiting to be energized. The yoga interpretation of the body has a basis in Western anatomy, too. According to physiology, both afferent and sensory nerves exist in the body:

➤ **Afferent nerves** carry messages to the brain and correspond to *pingala*.

➤ **Sensory nerves** carry messages from the brain to the rest of the body and correspond to *ida*.

The spinal cord or center of these two currents (afferent/*pingala* and sensory/*ida*), *sushumna,* also controls the currents that move through the body's nervous system. In yoga, there are 10 currents, called *nadis*. *Pingala, ida,* and *sushumna* are the major three.

Picturing the physiology (Western-style!) of your thoracic cavity (the cavity containing your lungs and heart) may help you visualize what's happening as you breathe during *pranayama*. When you inhale, your 24 ribs and two lungs expand. Your diaphragm, a large, flat muscle at the base of your thoracic cavity, moves

Know Your Sanskrit

Pingala (pronounced *pin-GAH-lah*) is a channel on the right side of the spine through which *prana* moves. ***Ida*** (*EE-dah*) is a channel on the left side of the spine through which *prana* moves. ***Sushumna*** (*soo-SHOOM-nah*) is a hollow passageway between *pingala* and *ida* that runs through the spinal cord, through which *kundalini* can travel once it's awakened. ***Nadis*** (*NAH-deez*) are psychospiritual energy pathways.

downward to make room for air rushing in. Imagine that it looks a little like an upside-down plunger, helping to pull air in. Deep breathing means filling your lungs from the bottom up. You have a lot of room in there for air!

The diaphragm muscle moves downward on inhalation and upward on exhalation. Take a deep breath and feel the muscle in motion!

When you exhale, your ribs and lungs contract. Your diaphragm rises, pushing the air back out, again like a plunger. When you breathe, imagine the breath is flowing deep into your abdomen, then slowly filling up the abdominal cavity, lower thoracic cavity, and last of all, the chest. On the exhalation, imagine the air flowing out from the chest, the lungs, past the diaphragm, and out of the deepest regions of the abdomen. This is deep breathing!

Try not to move your chest or shoulders when you breathe. All movement should be in your abdomen or lower rib area. Put your hand on your abdomen and try to expand and contract from there. And keep those shoulders still! Rising and falling shoulders are usually an indication of shallow breathing.

Wise Yogi Tells Us

According to wise *yogis*, the length of life is a matter of the number of breaths, not the number of years. Breath is so important to an accomplished *yogi* that he or she can get almost all necessary energy from the air. Sleeping? Eating? Minor concerns compared to the breath! That's why *yogis* have been known to sleep for just a few hours a night. All their energy is replenished through *pranayama* instead—the *yogi*'s beauty sleep!

Breath Control Equals Mental Control

Your breath and your mind have an intimate relationship. Just think about all the ways your breath is affected purely because your mind is experiencing something completely unrelated to breathing. Spend an entire day tuning in to your breath. Notice how it quickens or slows according to what you're doing, saying, or even thinking? Your breath can be affected merely by who you're near.

Just imagine watching an exciting movie. You're sitting still in your seat eating your popcorn. You aren't doing anything at all to get out of breath. As the opening credits roll, you see the name of your favorite actor or actress and your breath quickens in anticipation. When the movie gets suspenseful, you hold your breath. When the action speeds up, so does your breathing. Your breath responds to the movie's happy ending by becoming steady, smooth, and regular. As the credits roll, if the movie was a satisfying experience, you may even feel winded, as if you had been through a workout.

What our brain perceives, our breath mirrors and our body experiences. Imagine harnessing this power! Just as the mind influences the breath and body, so can the breath influence the mind and body. Controlling the power of breath is the technique of *pranayama*.

There are actually five manifestations of *prana* that act as vital energy in the body, depending on where they are. Each type complements one of the five nerve centers and is associated with one of the body's primary energy centers or, *chakras* (see Chapter 20, "*Chakras, Mudras, Mantras,* and *Mandalas,*" for more on *chakras*):

➤ *Prana* (PRAH-nah)—not the *prana* that is the universal life force, but a sort of "sub-*prana*"—rules the respiration process. It manifests in the heart *chakra* in the chest, flows into the body through inhalation, and moves up toward the brain.

➤ *Apana* (ah-PAH-nah) controls excretion, including the kidney, bladder, colon, genitals, and rectum. It's generated in the body by exhalation and flows downward toward the rectum and out of the body, ridding the body of impurities. It manifests through the Saturn *chakra* in the lower abdomen.

➤ *Samana* (sah-MAH-nah) governs the digestive system, including the stomach, intestine, liver, and pancreas. It manifests through the Mars *chakra* behind the stomach.

➤ *Udana* (uh-DAH-nah) lives in the throat and controls swallowing. It also serves as the force dividing the astral body (the vehicle of the spirit) from the physical body at the time of death. It's the vital energy of speech and manifests through the Mercury *chakra* in the throat.

➤ *Vyana* (vee-AH-nah) flows throughout the entire body, regulating blood flow as well as muscle and joint movements. It's the vital energy of circulation and manifests through the Jupiter *chakra* located on the spine near the genitals.

What does all this mean for you? In short, the more *prana* you bring into your body, the better your body and your mind will work, and the better you'll feel. *Prana* gives you instant energy and supports long-term good health. It is the ultimate feel-good medicine and a powerful preventive healthcare tool.

Blow Your Mind

So how do you get that *prana* inside you where it belongs? By learning *pranayama,* or yoga breathing techniques. *Pranayama* isn't difficult, but it takes concentration. There are many exercises to try. Following are a few. Experiment with each and consider incorporating a few of them into your yoga workout, between poses, before or after your workout, or whenever you need instant energy or calming.

You can practice breathing exercises just about anywhere, but they'll be more productive if you practice them in certain positions. All the following exercises will work better when your spine is aligned and your lungs are able to expand to their maximum, not when you're slumped over in a chair watching television. Let your body position make things simpler.

For each of the exercises, sit with your spine straight, on the floor or in a chair. Or choose one of the meditative postures from Chapter 17, "Are You Sitting Down?"

Om *Exhalation*

This technique extends the breath, softens it, and makes quieting the mind easier. Soon you'll feel a oneness drawing you closer to *samadhi.*

1. Inhale deeply, imagining your breath is moving all the way to the root of your spine.

2. Open your lips and begin to make the *Om* sound while exhaling slowly. "Ooooooooooooommmmmmmm," spending approximately 20 seconds on the "Oh" sound and about 10 seconds on the "mmm" sound.

3. Feel as if your entire being is enveloped in the sound. Let it surround and fill you.

4. Repeat several times.

Ujjayi: *Drawing Breath*

Jaya means "success on the spiritual path," and *ujjayi* means "she who is victorious." The *ujjayi* (pronounced *oo-JAH-yee*) technique aids in recalling and working with your dreams. It is also cooling to the head, aids digestion, soothes nerves, and tones the body. This breathing exercise produces sound in the throat with the inhalation.

1. Inhale slowly, keeping the lips closed and closing off the glottis, which is the opening between the vocal chords. Make a soft, humming sound: "hahhhh-hhh." Think Darth Vader breathing.

2. Imagine you are inhaling all the way to your heart. The upper portion of your lungs is full. You should feel the passage of the exhale, and you should hear it from the roof of your mouth.

3. Repeat several times.

Bhastrika: *Bellows Breath*

Bhastrika (pronounced *bah-STREE-kah*) is a powerful technique. Progress with it slowly to make the foundation strong. The bellows breath brings heat to the body and is excellent for weight reduction. It clears energy, purifies the physical body, and opens up restrictions in the spine, permitting a freer energy flow.

Bhastrika: *bellows breath.*

1. Exhale deeply and sharply, feeling your diaphragm muscle (refer to our definition earlier in this chapter) pull your navel in.

2. Inhale and exhale rapidly through your nose by continuing to force air out with sharp movements of your diaphragm. Don't worry about the inhale, which will take care of itself. Concentrate on the force of the exhalations.

3. Don't hold your breath between breaths. Aim for deep, quick movements of the diaphragm muscle. Remember, the inhalation will take little effort, especially as you practice this exercise and feel how the inhalation is a natural reflex following the exhalation.

4. Do 10 cycles, then hold your breath for a few seconds.

5. Repeat as many times as possible. If the strength of your exhalation begins to weaken, reduce the number of breaths in a cycle.

Kapalabhati: *Skull Shining*

A Yoga Minute

We inhale oxygen and exhale carbon dioxide. Trees and plants inhale carbon dioxide and exhale oxygen. Perfect harmony!

Kapalabhati (pronounced *KAH-pah-lah-BAH-tee*), or skull shining, is similar to bellows breath, but with a slow inhalation and a strong exhalation, and with a pause after each exhalation. This exercise has similar benefits but is like a calmer, easier, slower version. It is therefore more calming than bellows breath, which is more energizing. Since the skull consists of sinus passages, the technique is called skull shining, because it shines or clears the sinuses. It is also said to make your nose prettier!

1. Feel your diaphragm muscle pull your navel in as you exhale deeply and sharply. Then pause, holding your breath, after the exhalation for just a second or two.

2. Inhale slowly and deeply, then exhale sharply again, forcing the air out as you did before. Again, pause after the exhalation for a few seconds.

3. Pause between cycles. Do as many cycles as you can, spending one minute on each cycle. Gradually increase the time of your meditation after the cycle.

Shitali: *Cooling Breath*

Shitali (pronounced *shee-TAH-lee*) is great for summer! This technique is healing to the body and cools it from excessive heat. It clears the eyes and ears, satisfies hunger and thirst, activates the liver, and improves digestion. *Shitali* involves rolling the tongue, then inhaling through it like a straw.

1. Roll your tongue into a tube and keep the tip of it slightly outside the mouth. (If you can't roll your tongue, just try to raise the sides as well as you can, or just stick it out!)

2. Draw in breath through your curled tongue as if you're sipping through a straw. Fill your lungs.

3. When your lungs are full, bring your tongue into your mouth and close your mouth.

4. Lower your chin slightly and retain the breath for a few seconds.

A Yoga Minute

Although tongue rolling has always been considered a simple, inherited genetic trait, recent evidence suggests otherwise. Many studies of identical twins have found that only one of the twins was able to roll his or her tongue. Some who couldn't roll their tongues have been able to learn how. In general, however, tongue rolling *is* easy for some and virtually impossible for others.

Wise Yogi Tells Us

Adults breathe an average of 16,000 quarts of air each day. According to *yogic* thought, your life is measured by breaths, so lengthening each breath lengthens your life.

5. Exhale slowly through your nose.

6. Repeat several times.

Bhramari: *Bee Breath*

Bhramari (pronounced brah-MAH-ree) is good for insomnia. It imitates the sound of a bee and literally means "she who roams" (as a bee roams). Energetically, it helps awaken *kundalini* energy. You'll make the soft, humming sound of a bee with this technique.

1. Sit in one of the meditative postures in Chapter 17 or comfortably in a chair or cross-legged on the floor. Close your eyes.

2. Close off your right nostril with your right thumb. Inhale through your left nostril.

3. Fill your lungs, close both nostrils, and retain your breath for a few seconds.

4. Open your left nostril and slowly exhale through the left nostril using your throat to make a soft "eeee" sound through your exhalation.

5. Keep the exhalation going as long as possible. Alternate nostrils.

6. Repeat, starting with the left nostril for the inhalation.

7. Gradually intensify the breath and increase the sound of the "eeee" (the bee is getting closer!).

8. Repeat several times, alternating nostrils.

Nadi Shodhana: *Alternate Nostril Breathing*

Nadi shodhana (pronounced *NAH-dee shoh-DAH-nah*) balances the male/female or *ha/tha* within. This means it balances the emotional and physical natures. For example, when your emotions become overwhelming, this technique brings you back to a balanced state. Gradually, the amount of time when both nostrils are closed should increase comfortably. Keep your finger movement to a minimum.

Finger position for nadi shodhana.

1. Sit in one of the meditative postures in Chapter 17, or comfortably in a chair or cross-legged on the floor. Close your eyes.

2. Cover your right nostril with your right thumb exhale. Inhale through your left nostril.

3. Close your left nostril with the ring finger of your right hand. Your two middle fingers should be turned in toward your palm.

4. Hold both nostrils closed for as long as you can comfortably. Then release the right nostril and exhale through it.

5. Inhale through your right nostril, then close it again.

6. Hold both nostrils closed for as long as you can comfortably. Then exhale through your left nostril.

7. Inhale through your left nostril, close, exhale through your right nostril, and so on.

8. Repeat several times.

Murccha Kumbhaka: *Third-Eye Breathing*

Murccha kumbhaka (pronounced *MER-chah koom-BHAH-kah*) focuses all your attention and energy on your third eye, which is the *chakra*, or energy center, located between and just above your eyebrows on your forehead. (For more on this and other *chakras*, see Chapter 20. This exercise produces a focused, blissful feeling.

1. Gently and slowly inhale, then hold your breath.

2. As you hold your breath, concentrate on the spot on your forehead about an inch above the place exactly between your eyebrows, called the third eye.

3. Hold your breath for as long as is comfortable, while staying focused on the third eye.

4. Exhale very slowly through your mouth, staying focused on the third eye.

5. Repeat several times.

Ouch!

Just as you shouldn't push your body to achieve a difficult posture before it's ready, you also need to be aware of your breath capacity. Don't practice one-minute inhalations and two-minute exhalations your first time out! You may faint or hyperventilate. As always, listen to your body. It will tell you when you're going too far. Go slowly.

Kevali Kumbhaka: *Hold Your Breath (But Not 'Til You Turn Blue!)*

Just like anything else, breath control and capacity increase with practice. In *kevali kumbhaka* (pronounced *kay-VAH-lee koom-BAH-kah*), you practice holding your breath. Don't make yourself dizzy. Don't hold your breath until you faint. Just hold your breath until you feel like you need to let it go again. The more you practice this technique, the longer you'll be able to hold your breath, which increases your lung capacity and makes your breathing more efficient.

1. Inhale deeply through the nose, then hold your breath.

2. Hold for as long as is comfortable.

3. Exhale gently, slowly, and fully.

4. Repeat several times.

We're confident you're feeling more energized by now. What a great way to prime your body for yoga postures—and life!

The Least You Need to Know

➤ *Prana* is the universal life force that permeates and animates everything, including you.

➤ *Prana* flows into the body via the breath, so controlling the breath controls the flow of *prana*.

➤ *Pranayama* are breathing techniques that, when practiced, result in better control of the mind and body.

➤ Practice *pranayama* with good posture for optimal results.

Chapter 8

Hatha Yoga: May the Force Be with You

Yoga's ultimate realization of self-actualization isn't so mystical. It is a practical path with concrete steps. What is self-actualization? Yoga books often talk about enlightenment, but modern Western psychology has a similar notion.

What Do We Need? East Meets West!

According to psychologist Abraham Maslow, humans have certain needs, from basic to fully evolved, that must be met for self-actualization to happen. These needs must be met approximately in order, because humans won't feel the "higher" needs until the "lower" needs are taken care of. Often represented in a pyramid graphic (looks a little like triangle pose in Chapter 13, "What Do You Stand For?"), Maslow's Hierarchy of Needs includes the following levels:

➤ First, our basic needs must be met: hunger, thirst, shelter, and physical comfort.

➤ Next, we must feel safe and out of danger.

➤ Third, according to Maslow, we require a sense of belonging and love. We need to know we are accepted and affiliated with others.

➤ Next, we need to achieve something, feel competent, gain approval, and develop a sense of self-esteem.

➤ Fifth comes the need to know and understand the world around us and ourselves.

➤ Sixth is our need to experience beauty and order, and to develop an aesthetic sense.

➤ Seventh is Maslow's level of self-actualization. Once our other needs are met, we experience a desire to find self-fulfillment, to realize our human potential, and to engage in work that is meaningful and to which we feel a personal calling.

➤ The last level of Maslow's Hierarchy of Needs is transcendence. Once we have found personal fulfillment, we can reach out to help others realize their human potential, too.

Maslow's Hierarchy of Needs.

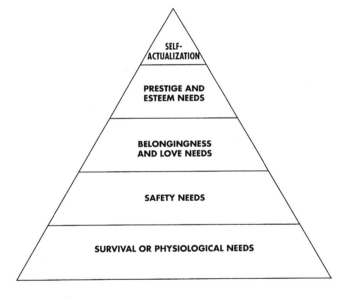

So where does yoga come in? *Hatha Yoga* is a yoga system that emphasizes the physical along the path of self-actualization. After our basic needs are met, we feel safe, and we feel loved, yoga comes into play.

The yoga path helps us control and train our minds so we are better able to embark on a cognitive search. Its order, balance, symmetry, and the beauty of the poses can help fulfill our desire for aesthetic experiences. It can serve as a mode for self-actualization, and it certainly contributes to fulfillment, to reaching individual human potential, to simplification; in short, to becoming fully realized human beings.

While yoga doesn't necessarily have to be the vocation or activity you choose for self-actualization (perhaps you are an artist, a writer, an entrepreneur, a scientist, whatever), yoga trains your body, your mind, and your spirit so you can learn the fine arts of concentration, focus, commitment, and total immersion in the activities of your life. And that's where self-actualization happens.

Self-actualization through yoga comes out of more than just the poses, or *asanas*. It comes from purifying body and mind to make room for new experiences and broader awareness. It comes from the discipline of personal hygiene and maintaining a clean, simple environment (yoga cleansing rituals are called *shodhana*). It comes from the vitalization of *pranayama* techniques (discussed in Chapter 7, "Can You Breathe?"). And it comes from the mental uncluttering of meditation.

Know Thyself

What does self-actualization or self-awareness mean to you? Self-awareness means different things to different people, but here are some ways to look at self-awareness. Self-awareness is …

➤ Finding out that the alignment of your large toe is responsible for your headache. Discovering that your body is full of links, clues, and connections to your health and mental well-being.

➤ Pausing before your emotions take over your actions, and eventually finding out that your emotions can exist without taking over.

➤ Feeling truly connected to another living thing—a parent, a child, a friend, a stranger in need, that stray cat that keeps hanging around.

➤ Breathing deeply and slowly; noticing how different that feels.

➤ Looking in the mirror and seeing beyond your reflection; seeing the inner you written all over your face.

➤ Having vision and direction in your life; finding a deeper calling and heeding it.

➤ Recognizing that the sun salutation (see Chapter 16, "A Continuous Flow") is reflective of the ebb and flow of life; finding the connection every day.

➤ Finding the clear steadiness of the eyes in an externally changing face; both inner and outer movement are ever possible.

➤ Experiencing pure joy simply by looking at something beautiful; you don't need to own it. You can be with it, then let it go.

➤ Finding inner peace. *Om.*

When the body is strong, controlled, and purified, *kundalini* energy can move freely up the spine and through the *chakras* without getting blocked anywhere along the way. (See Chapter 20, "*Chakras, Mudras, Mantras,* and *Mandalas.*") If *kundalini* energy gets blocked, both physical and mental problems could result. The body that's physically prepared for the rise of *kundalini* energy will derive the ultimate benefit from its power. *Hatha Yoga* is that physical preparation.

Joining the Sun and the Moon

Hatha Yoga is about balancing the opposing forces of the body, just as opposing forces are balanced outside of the body. Sun and moon, male and female, day and night, cold and hot—the universe is filled with opposites. Maybe you've heard of or seen the yin/yang symbol. This ancient Chinese symbol (see the following illustration) represents the universe of opposing forces. Notice how a white dot sits in the center of the black swirl, and a black dot sits in the center of the white swirl.

The yin/yang union.

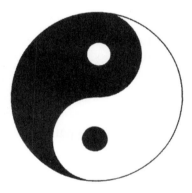

Yin and yang are commonly associated with many different complementary qualities. Yin is primarily present in the moon, the night, cold, female energy, and heaviness. Yang is primarily present in the sun, the daytime, heat, male energy, and lightness. And since every force has an opposite, and also contains a bit of its opposite within, male energy contains female energy, female energy contains male energy, night contains a bit of day in it, day a bit of night, and so on. So the universe goes—ultimately interconnected.

And so our bodies go, too. We are filled with opposites: a left and a right side, blood flowing to the heart and away from the heart, the delivery of nutrients and the removal of waste, our inhalations and exhalations, our hunger and satiety, sleeping and wakefulness, being with others and being alone, joy and sadness, birth and death, growth and decline. If any of the thousands of opposites and intricate balances within us become unbalanced, our bodies and minds won't work as efficiently.

Hatha Yoga balances us in many ways. Forward-bending postures are followed by backbending postures, contractions are followed by extensions, upright positions are followed by inversions, and so on. The practice of *Hatha Yoga* also balances our mental and spiritual energies—for what we do with the body affects the mind and the spirit (that triangle again!). Ultimately interconnected.

On a subtler level, the movement of *prana* is balanced through muscular exercises called *bandhas*. As *prana* is drawn into the body through the inhalation of breath, *apana* is the energy generated in the body by exhalation that moves away from the brain and carries impurities out of the body. *Bandhas* are exercises, or muscular locks, designed to lock the flow of energy in the body.

The three primary *bandhas* are …

> ➤ At the chin (called *jalandhara bandha*). This *bandha* strengthens and builds *prana*'s upward movement by bringing the chin to the chest.

> ➤ In the pelvis (called *uddiyana bandha*). This *bandha* strengthens and builds *apana*'s downward movement by pulling your navel up and back toward your spine.

> ➤ In the area of the rectum (called *mula bandha*). This *bandha* keeps *prana* from escaping from the lower body by contracting the perineal muscle (the muscle you sit on, in front of the rectum).

Know Your Sanskrit

Apana is the energy generated in the body by exhalation that moves away from the brain and carries impurities out of the body. *Bandha* means "to bind" or "to lock," and *bandhas* are muscular locks used during postures and breathing exercises to intensify the energy of *prana* and *apana* so it can eliminate impurities from the body. The three primary *bandhas* are anal **ormula bandha** (MOO-lah BAHN-dah), stomach or **uddiyani bandha** (ooh-dee-YAH-nah BAHN-dah), and chin or **jalandhara bandha** (jah-lahn-DAH-rah BAHN-dah).

Bandhas keep the system of balances in check by pulling everything toward a center point, intensifying the energy. Practicing these *bandhas* together while sitting in a meditative pose such as the lotus pose is a particularly powerful technique for concentrating and intensifying *prana* in the body.

Practicing the bandhas.

A Yoga Minute

In Hindu culture, cobras are considered reincarnations of important people. The Aztecs worshipped a snake god who symbolized light, luck, and wisdom. In Africa, some cultures worship pythons, and killing snakes is a crime. Egyptian kings wore snake representations on their crowns, and the crosier of *Asklepios* (the Greek god of medicine and healing) is still a symbol of the medical profession.

The result is that *prana* and *apana* are retained within the body, joining together within *sushumna*—that hollow passageway through your spinal cord. Their mingling generates an intense energy that can help awaken the *kundalini* serpent power. This joining of opposites, of *prana* and *apana,* of sun and moon, of *ha* and *tha,* is at the heart of *Hatha Yoga*'s power. Maybe you aren't too concerned with awakening your serpent power, especially since you aren't too sure exactly what it is—or even whether you want to know. Maybe you just want to feel more balanced, healthier, more in shape. Most Westerners don't practice *Hatha Yoga* to the extent that they're even aware of the importance of *kundalini* energy, but traditionally, this awakening of the "serpent power" is one of the primary purposes of *Hatha Yoga.*

Physical fitness—making the body feel good and look good—has traditionally been a peripheral benefit, but it has shifted to the primary focus for Westerners. If fitness is your motivation for beginning a *Hatha Yoga* practice, that's great. You'll benefit in many ways, no matter what reason brings you to the practice. But while fitness is important in *Hatha Yoga,* it means more than cut shoulders and washboard abs. Total fitness—of the mind, body, and spirit—is a far cry from body obsession. Body obsession is fitness gone awry.

If fitness is your goal, it doesn't hurt (and may even be ultimately helpful) to be aware of the power of balanced opposites inherent in your practice. This knowledge may steer you away from the path of body glorification—a possible side effect of heightened body awareness—and toward the more advanced paths of mental control (*Raja Yoga*) and spiritual awakening.

Hatha Yoga *joins the opposites of sun and moon within the body. Here the energies are drawn into the centered position of respect and thanks,* namaste, *or prayer pose.*

Training the Body to Free the Mind

Think how much time you spend worrying about your body! Check all the following statements that have ever crossed your mind:

❑ I'm too fat.

❑ I'm too thin.

❏ I'm having a bad hair day.

❏ My skin looks terrible.

❏ My body is unattractive.

❏ I have the best body in the room.

Our bodies are so much a part of us and so emphasized by our culture that it's extremely difficult not to put too much emphasis on physical appearance. Remember, though, that your body isn't all of you. In fact, your body is just one tiny part of you. You are the entire universe. You have the potential for perfection, contentment, and pure joy. Your body is just a convenient container for the luminous being that is you. In comparison to who you really are, even the most "perfect" body is a little, well … crude?

Wise Yogi Tells Us

Once you're comfortable in some of the postures, try adding a new dimension to your workout: visualization. Visualization is the process of picturing something in your mind and letting it affect you. Visualizing something beautiful—an ocean, a sparkling lake, a magnificent canyon, a spectacular sunset—can make you feel peaceful and relaxed. Practice visualization while holding postures that are easy for you. Hold your image for as long as you can before other thoughts take over.

One Body … or Three?

You have one body—or do you? Actually, according to yoga, you have three bodies: the physical body, the astral body, and the causal body. These three bodies can function separately, but they are intimately interrelated, too.

Maintaining an awareness of all three of your bodies will help you see more clearly who you really are. Self-actualization means knowing your *whole* self.

Here's a closer look at your three bodies:

➤ The *physical* body is the crudest of the bodies and the smallest. This is the you in the mirror. Yet even though it's crude, it's our best tool for growth. We can't deny we have physical bodies, so yoga helps us make the most of them. The first three aspects of Patanjali's Eightfold Path strengthen and train the physical body: abstinences (*yamas*), observances (*niyamas*), and postures (*asanas*). (See Chapter 6, "Walking Yoga's Eightfold Path.")

➤ The *astral* body is the vehicle of the spirit and corresponds with the mind. This layer exists within the causal body and encompasses the physical body. It is like layer number two, the second layer to form, extending beyond the physical body but not to the limits of the causal body. The astral body is strengthened through the next three steps of the Eightfold Path: breathing exercises (*pranayama*), sense withdrawal (*pratyahara*), and concentration (*dharana*).

➤ The *causal* body is the largest, most widely reaching layer of you, starting with spirit. It's the subtlest body and holds the spirit, as well as the other layers. This is where you started. Individuality (as we normally think of it) exists to a minimal degree in the causal body, which allows the spirit to shine and truth to be evident. The causal body is reached or experienced through the final two limbs of the Eightfold Path: meditation (*dhyana*) and superconsciousness or bliss (*samadhi*).

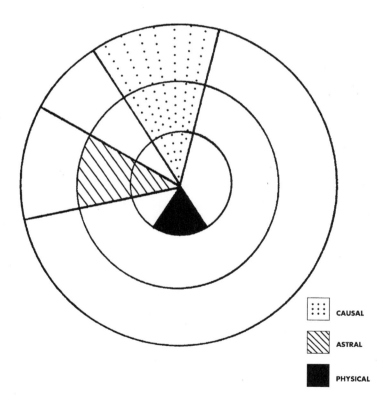

You have three interpenetrating bodies—yes, you! These are the physical, causal, and astral bodies.

⋮⋮⋮ **CAUSAL**

▨ **ASTRAL**

■ **PHYSICAL**

Hatha Yoga works under the assumption that the inner you is the you worth working on, but to get to the inner you, the outer you—in all its crudity—must first be controlled. *Hatha Yoga* works to get the physical body under control and in balance so it doesn't impede the other bodies—the astral and causal. Only then can the self-actualized, balanced you emerge in your full glory.

Hatha Yoga accomplishes this Herculean task of fine-tuning and delicate balancing by ...

➤ Building strength through exercises.

➤ Toning the organs and joints through exercises.

➤ Training the breath.

➤ Keeping the body infused with *prana*.

➤ Keeping the body clean.

Through these exercises, techniques, and rituals, the body is properly prepared for the rising of *kundalini* energy.

Hatha Yoga is about balance and emphasizes *pranayama* and *asanas,* or postures. *Raja Yoga*, or royal path, also incorporates Patanjali's Eightfold Path, but with a greater emphasis on sense withdrawal, concentration, and meditation. *Hatha* and *Raja Yoga* exist in a symbiotic relationship. If you've mastered your body and your breath so that *prana* is able to flow freely and unencumbered through your *chakras,* meditation is the natural next step in the progression. You have prepared your body to optimize meditation. In turn, meditation prepares your mind to stand back and let the spirit shine through.

As you look in the mirror, you might wonder about those different levels, those three bodies, and what they really are to the reflection you see. Actually, within the three bodies, there are five sheaths of existence, according to yoga. What you see in the mirror is only one of those sheaths, or *koshas* (which can be translated as "envelopes") that make up the real you.

Know Your Sanskrit

Koshas (pronounced *KOH-shahs*) are the five sheaths of existence that make up the body: the physical body, the vital body, the mind sheath, the intellect sheath, and the sheath of bliss.

The Physical

➤ The physical body, *anna-maya-kosha* (pronounced *AH-nah MAI-ah KOH-shah*) or "food envelope," consists of your material body. This is what you see in the mirror.

➤ The vital body, *prana-maya-kosha* (pronounced *PRAH-nah MAI-ah KOH-shah*), is where *prana* lives and moves. It exists just beyond your physical body; it's your aura.

The Emotional or Astral

➤ The mind sheath, *mano-maya-kosha* (pronounced *MAH-noh MAI-ah KOH-shah*), is the seat of the part of your mind that interprets all sensory input. "I have an awareness of an emotion."

➤ The intellect sheath, *vijnana-maya-kosha* (pronounced *vizh-NAH-nah MAI-ah KOH-shah*), houses your intelligence and wisdom. "I am aware that I am more than my emotions."

The Causal (Where Everything Starts)

➤ The bliss sheath, *ananda-maya-kosha* (pronounced *ah-NAHN-dah MAI-ah KOH-shah*), contains the field of energy that links you with the universe and in which all is bliss. This was the source of the original you, the other sheaths are unfolding all the way down into an incarnation—again, that's you in the mirror.

Did you have any idea you were walking around with all those layers?

Physical Cleansing

But what's all this about keeping the body so clean? You take showers. You wash your hair. You use deodorant. You don't smell bad. Isn't that enough? Not to the *yogi!* Of course, nothing should become an obsession, but to Hindu culture, where yoga has its roots, the body is impure and needs some serious hygienic upkeep to keep it from becoming a hindrance to the spirit and an impediment to *kundalini* energy.

This cleanliness is called *shodhana* and consists of cleansing rituals, *shat kriyas,* for the body. *Hatha Yoga* also concerns strict observance of dental hygiene. *Yogis* not only brush their teeth but rinse their mouths, massage their gums, and scrape their tongues to keep them clean. And don't forget to visit your dentist every six months! (If you follow that *yogi* regimen, your dentist will be very impressed.)

Read on for more on some of the other *shat kriyas.*

Know Your Sanskrit

Shat kriyas (pronounced *SHOT kree-yahs*) are the purification rituals of *Hatha Yoga.* **Shodhana** (*sho-DAH-nah*) is purification of the body.

Sthala Basti (Ground Colon Cleansing): Elimination Illumination!

Let's start at the bottom. This ritual helps relieve gas and keeps the bowels moving smoothly. It also improves the digestion and gives your body a lighter feel.

Sit with your legs stretched out in front of you. Grab your toes, right toe with your right hand, left toe with your left hand. Bend forward, bringing your head toward your knees just a little, so that it feels comfortable. Relax the abdominal muscles, then churn them up and down. While churning your muscles, "lock" your anus (this is the *mula bandha,* one of the three *bandhas* discussed earlier in this chapter). Be very careful not to push yourself too hard. This ritual should feel comfortable. Practice this ritual on an empty stomach, or drink a glass of pure water first.

Agnisara Dhauti (Fire Stomach Cleansing): Tummy Toner

This ritual is called Fire Stomach Cleansing because it stokes the gastric fire and improves digestion. It helps keep the bowels healthy, cures constipation, and reduces belly fat. If you have abdominal problems or circulatory problems, you should avoid this cleansing ritual.

Perform this ritual by squatting just slightly from a standing position with your legs about one foot apart or slightly more. Exhale fully, then hold your breath. Next, perform the muscle churning described in the Ground Colon Cleansing ritual, but with the stomach muscles, moving them in more of a circular motion than an up-and-down motion. Rotate the muscles in this way as quickly as you can for as long as you can without discomfort. Don't push to the point where you become exhausted.

After the muscle churning, relax and let the breath flow in and out. This makes one round. Work up to several rounds, eventually reaching 100 or so churning rotations.

Wise Yogi Tells Us

If all these cleansing rituals seem like a little much to you, keep in mind that they are ancient Hindu practices based in a culture that considers the body ultimately earthy. Practice good hygiene to whatever degree makes you comfortable.

Kapalabhati: Blow Off Some Steam

Kapalabhati (pronounced *KAH-pah-lah-BAH-tee*) is both a cleansing ritual and a breathing exercise. Remember it from the last chapter? *Kapalabhati* is the "Skull Shining" *pranayama* technique with the slow inhale and the sharp exhale meant to cleanse the respiratory passages and lungs. (See a more detailed description in

Chapter 7.) It is often included as a part of *pranayama* practice. This cleansing breath clears the sinuses, improves circulation, and charges your bloodstream with oxygen. It's said to increase longevity and prepare the body for the practice of *pranayama*.

Neti: *Bless You!*

Neti (pronounced *NAY-tee*) involves various methods for cleansing the nasal passages. One method is to sniff water into the nostrils and spit it out of the mouth, called *vuyt-krama* (*VOOT KRAY-mah*)—but please don't drown yourself! The water should be neither hot nor cold. You can also buy *neti* bottles; you use these to pour water into one nostril, which will then come out the other nostril. We prefer to simply blow our noses when necessary and suggest this might be the best course for you, too. *Neti* is good for relieving nasal congestion or even putting the brakes on an allergy attack.

Trataka: *Seeing the Light*

Trataka (pronounced *trah-TAH-kah*) cleanses the eyes by focusing them on a candle flame until they start to water. Gaze at a candle flame from a distance of at least two feet (don't bring your eyes too close to the candle). After a few minutes, rinse your eyes in cold water. *Trataka* is said to strengthen the eyes and, in some cases, induce *clairvoyance*. It can also be used as a meditation technique, with the candle flame as a point of focus.

Stabilizing the Body's Energies

You may be eager to hear a little more about the aspect of *Hatha Yoga* many Westerners consider the most interesting. Yes, the *asanas,* or yoga poses, are very important to the practice of *Hatha Yoga,* but not because yoga's purpose is to make you look great in a bathing suit or allow you to flaunt your flexibility.

In fact, even as we say that *Hatha Yoga's* emphasis is on the physical, we really mean *Hatha Yoga* emphasizes the physical in order to, eventually, *de*emphasize the physical. Once you've mastered control of your body—once you're strong, flexible, and "master of your domain"—you can forget about your body!

In the state of *samadhi,* the self, including the body, blends into the universal energy we are all part of. All that body work is really just a way to learn how to transcend your body! And that will make your yoga journey easier.

A Yoga Minute

Perform each cleansing ritual in the spirit of loving devotion, always keeping nonviolence (*ahimsa*) in mind.

Think of it this way: All your life, you've wanted to live in Florida, or Alaska, or California, or wherever. But you live on the opposite side of the country—say, in Providence, Rhode Island; or Amarillo, Texas. Finally, you're ready to start your big move, so you purchase a really nice car for your journey. As you drive across the country, you do everything you can to keep your car in top condition so you won't have any breakdowns or mechanical failures. You learn all about your car so you know what you're driving. And sure enough, you get there without a hitch, or if a tire blows out or a belt breaks, you know exactly what to do.

Hatha Yoga is the same way. The idea is not the car, or the body, but the destination and finding joy along the way. You want to get to Florida, and you know the best way to get there is to have a vehicle in great condition. Keep your body in great condition. Know your body. Know yourself. You'll be less likely to wind up in the shop (the doctor's office) for repairs!

Achieving Vitality

Pranayama is the final, crucial aspect of *Hatha Yoga* all *yogis* will do well to practice. We talk about *pranayama* in detail in Chapter 7, so we'll just say a few more words here about *prana* and vitality.

Prana is vitality. Mastering *prana,* both physical and mental, is probably the single most important aspect of *Hatha Yoga. Prana* powers the universe with its energy, and it's the profound connection between you and everything else. Amazingly, something as simple as a breathing technique is the first step to becoming aware of the movement of *prana* through your body and throughout the universe.

Even though *prana* can't be measured or observed, it can certainly be sensed by the *yogi* tuned in to its power. Wise *yogis* and others throughout history perceive *prana* on an intuitive level; those who use it will be astonished at its power. Try a little *pranayama* today, and you, too, will be on your way to greater awareness. *Prana* happens!

The Least You Need to Know

➤ *Hatha Yoga* is a balance of opposing forces.

➤ A trained body won't get in the way of spiritual enlightenment and can even encourage it.

➤ Cleanliness is next to enlightenment.

➤ *Prana* is in you, animates you, and flows through the universe.

Part 3

Starting Your Yoga Practice

Here's your comprehensive guide to getting started. You'll learn how to find a yoga class and a good teacher, how to practice on your own at home, what to wear, when to practice, and how to fit yoga into your busy schedule. You'll also find tips for changing the way you think about exercise, from banishing the "no pain, no gain" adage from your mentality to learning how your breath can enhance your workout.

You'll have a chance to examine your motives and reasons for considering yoga by taking an essay test you can't fail. It will help to direct your thinking inward and allow you to better analyze your strengths and tendencies. Knowing your body and mind will help you craft a yoga routine that will work best for you.

Chapter 9

Where Do You Practice Yoga?

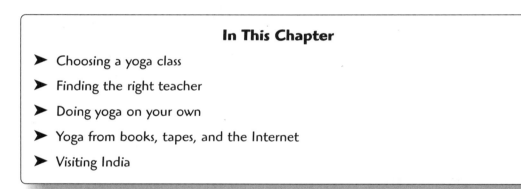

In This Chapter

➤ Choosing a yoga class

➤ Finding the right teacher

➤ Doing yoga on your own

➤ Yoga from books, tapes, and the Internet

➤ Visiting India

So you've decided to give yoga a try. Great! Now what? Now is the time to make a game plan. Decide how you would like to proceed with your yoga. Do you want to take a class and reap the benefits of a qualified instructor? Do you want to try yoga on your own for a while, then consider a class later if you like what you experience? Maybe you want to go all out and book passage to Calcutta!

Whatever course you choose to take, make sure you have the necessary preparation so you can get the most from your yoga experience. Your personality, your schedule, and your general inclinations will all have an effect on the type of yoga that will serve you most effectively.

Choosing a Yoga Class

Probably the best way to start out with yoga is to take a class. You can learn a lot from books and videos, but a real live teacher can address your personal challenges and direct you in ways a book can't. (But don't stop reading this book yet! We still have a lot left to tell you.) Consider the following reasons to take a yoga class:

➤ A teacher can see you from all angles, making minor adjustments in your posture to help you get the most from each position.

➤ A teacher can advise you on the best postures for your particular physical challenges, such as a stiff neck, lower back pain, or tennis elbow.

➤ If you have a class to attend at a prescheduled time, you may be less likely to put off or skip your practice. And regular exercise is the most beneficial for anyone.

➤ Other students learning yoga along with you can offer peer support and camaraderie, in addition to your teacher's encouragement.

➤ A class and a qualified teacher in conjunction with personal practice and lots of books on the subject will teach you more about yoga than any one of these methods alone.

A Yoga Minute

When you look for a yoga class, you have several factors to consider: the teacher's method and approach, the size of the class, class schedules, and so on. Plan to spend some time exploring the possibilities before you find the teacher and the class that suit your particular needs.

Yoga classes vary greatly in their format and approach, so if you do decide to take a class, you'll first want to do a bit of shopping. The right yoga class is highly personal—what *you* love, your friends may not benefit from at all, and vice versa. If you are used to a high-energy, aerobic workout, you may initially be impatient with yoga's slower pace, although it will serve as an excellent balance for your life. If you're generally inactive, you may benefit more from a yoga class where steady, flowing yoga movements get the heart pumping.

You also might be confused about the wide array of yoga methods. The difference is largely due to who has most directly influenced the teacher or under which method the teacher was trained. Before signing up for a class, ask the teacher which school of yoga he or she practices, and then ask him or her to explain the basic philosophy of that particular school or method.

Make sure any yoga class you consider meets the following criteria:

➤ The yoga teacher is a qualified instructor. Anyone can teach yoga—not everyone can teach it well. Don't be fooled by health clubs touting "yoga" classes taught by club employees who might have read a book on yoga or who think all fitness is basically the same. Some health clubs offer excellent yoga classes, but you'll want to ask about the teacher's training.

➤ The class is small enough that the teacher can give you individual attention. You'll want help adjusting postures and creating a routine suited to your ability so you won't get injured, frustrated, or bored silly.

➤ The class is conveniently scheduled and easy to get to. Otherwise, you know what will happen. Eventually, going to class will be too much trouble and it won't last.

If you don't like your first class, your first teacher, or the way you felt after your first yoga workout, don't give up. Some people overdo it their first time out and vow never to practice yoga again. If you can't relate to your teacher; if you pull a muscle; or if the class environment is high-pressure, competitive, or unpleasant in any way, you just haven't found the right class or the right teacher for you.

Or maybe you weren't completely open to the experience—could your competitive nature have overshadowed the benefits you were receiving? Was the teacher encouraging a competitive attitude, or was the teacher inattentive to your needs? Maybe you couldn't understand what the teacher wanted you to do. (Teachers are human, too.) Many teachers are grounded in the noncompetitive philosophy, but some still see yoga simply as physical fitness, with all its competitive aspects. Many are excellent at doling out individual help and counsel, but others may have classes that are too large for a really personal approach.

Wise Yogi Tells Us

Having trouble finding a yoga class? Try these sources:

➤ A natural foods/health store

➤ A health club or fitness center

➤ Your local hospital

➤ Your local university, college, or community college

➤ Local holistic health practitioners

Reflective pose.

The most important thing you can do for your yoga practice is to find a teacher you feel comfortable with, so keep looking until you find him or her. And remember what you have learned so far: Yoga is about fitness for and knowledge of your whole self, not just your body.

The bottom line? Be patient in your search. It may take a while to find the right class and the right teacher for you, but many *yogis* believe that when the student is ready, the right teacher will appear. Keep your mind and heart open.

Finding Your Personal *Guru*

You've heard the word, we're sure, but you may be confused as to what a *guru* actually is. A *guru* is a spiritual teacher. You can have many spiritual teachers in your life, but traditionally, you have only one *guru,* and you attach, spiritually, not only to the *guru* but to the *guru*'s lineage (in other words, the particular tradition out of which that *guru* comes, what he or she has studied, what "school" or "branch" of yoga he or she is associated with). Literally, the word *guru* means "dispeller of darkness," and that is the *guru*'s role: to help you dispel your own spiritual darkness.

Do you need a *guru?* Not necessarily. But perhaps. A *guru*/disciple relationship between mature individuals is really a journey of spiritual revelations and discoveries for both disciple and *guru.* The *guru*'s "job" is to give you spiritual guidance and insight, and to insist that you think for yourself. In fact, it is essential that a disciple have the freedom to follow or not follow that guidance. A good disciple will travel toward spiritual independence, but a *guru* makes a great traveling companion with an excellent road map to get you well on your way.

The concept of the *guru* is a little hard for us Westerners to swallow. After all, we like to be self-sufficient. We aren't a submissive, follow-the-leader type of culture, and the idea that we should surrender to some kind of a superior—putting our physical, mental, and spiritual development in his or her hands—makes us uncomfortable. This isn't a difficult concept for many Easterners, whose culture has taught them, over the course of centuries, that the best way to truly learn anything—a craft, a posture, a philosophy, enlightenment—is by loyal devotion to a wise individual who has sage advice and knowledge to impart.

We Westerners like to question, and our doubting natures are only encouraged when we hear story after story about spiritual teachers and leaders who have gone astray. Our modern world is full of temptations, and sometimes *gurus,* priests, evangelists, healers, and others whose purpose is to lead others to a higher spiritual plane cave in to temptation. A true, enlightened *guru* will remain your spiritual guide for a lifetime, but these days, good *gurus* are hard to find! (And many a *guru* will counter that good students are equally hard to find!)

But you may not need a *guru*—at least not in the traditional sense. For some, a *guru* is a crucial part of the yoga journey, but for others, a teacher is the perfect guide. A qualified yoga teacher you truly connect with can be your most valuable resource. A great yoga teacher can change your life and improve your practice of yoga far beyond what you could figure out on your own. And we all have a *guru* within. Most important, don't be discouraged if you haven't found the *acarya* or *guru* who is right for you. Be patient, keep your eyes open, keep practicing, don't be afraid to be picky, don't put up with mediocre instruction or a teacher who doesn't understand you, and eventually, if it's meant to work out that way, you'll find the perfect fit. Ultimately, the fit is an internal one.

Know Your Sanskrit

Acarya (pronounced *ah-CAHR-yah*) means "teacher."

Going Solo at Home

If you aren't quite ready for the commitment of a class, or if for any other reason you don't want to or aren't able to take a class, do-it-yourself yoga can be very rewarding. Design your own workout from the poses in this book (see Chapter 12, "Crafting Your Personalized Yoga Practice"), find a comfortable practice area, dress in comfortable clothing (see Chapter 10, "How to Practice Yoga"), designate a regular practice time (whether once a week or twice a day—we suggest daily), and get ready for your very first *asana!*

Setting Up Your Practice Area

One of the great things about yoga is that you can do it almost anywhere—in the bedroom, in the living room, even outside! Your environment should consistently include several things, however:

➤ **A soft surface.** Nonskid carpets are good surfaces for practicing yoga, but if your floor isn't carpeted or is slippery, use a small rug, a blanket, or a yoga mat (a thin rubber mat that can be placed on any surface for a comfortable, nonskid surface). You need the firmness of the ground, but the surface on which you work should be soft enough to be comfortable. If you practice outside, bring along a blanket or mat that can get a little dirty.

Ouch!

Keeping warm while practicing yoga is extremely important. If your muscles are cold, they can stiffen and lose flexibility, increasing your chance of injury. Warm muscles and joints are most conducive to a yoga workout. Also, in quieter poses and during meditation, you'll become colder more easily because you aren't encouraging active circulation.

➤ **A source of warmth.** In the summer, you probably won't have to worry about keeping warm, but in the winter or in a drafty room, warmth can be an issue. Keep a blanket nearby to drape around yourself during still poses, breathing exercises, and meditation. Your muscles need to be warm to stay flexible, and you need to be comfortable to get the most from your practice. Practicing outside in the sun on a warm day is ideal. If you practice inside in the winter, consider a small electric heater (please use it safely) for your practice area.

➤ **Fresh air.** If you practice inside and weather permits, open a window and take a few deep breaths of fresh air before you start. Practicing outside will, of course, immerse you in fresh air (unless you live in a polluted environment, in which case you are probably better off practicing inside). If the weather doesn't permit (if it's too cold or too hot outside), don't worry about the fresh air. You'll get some when the temperature is milder.

Practice in an area free of obstacles and distractions. Practicing yoga amid clutter and confusion is difficult and even counterproductive. As we've mentioned before, cleanliness is important to yoga, and that includes an uncluttered and clean environment. Although a seasoned *yogi* can find a sense of serenity in any setting (even your family room, where your teenager is playing video games and your twin toddlers are practicing for a career in large-building demolition), you may not be able to focus quite as well as you would in a quiet room all by yourself.

Even if the rest of your house is a perpetual disaster area, try to keep one special "yoga spot" clear, clean, pet-free, kid-free, and relatively quiet. Before you know it, the rest of your house will "magically" become less cluttered and more simply furnished. It's yet another positive influence yoga can have on your lifestyle.

Yoga from Tapes and Videos

Another great way to learn yoga is with a yoga videotape or audiotape. With a tape, you can see (or at least hear) a teacher. You can watch the postures performed or hear them described, which can be easier to follow than a static picture in a book. The teacher on the tape can offer advice and wisdom vocally. Some people comprehend information better if they see or hear it than if they read it, while others benefit much more from the written word.

If your teacher has made tapes or videos, you can use them to extend your in-person yoga practice by taking your teacher home with you via electronic media. Taking advantage of all possible levels of study will result in more learning opportunities.

Wise Yogi Tells Us

When practicing postures at home on your own, it may help to keep in mind these five steps to every pose:

➤ Visualize your body holding the pose.

➤ Gracefully flow into the pose.

➤ Become one with the pose—find the peace and balance.

➤ Gracefully flow out of the pose.

➤ Reflect and release. Let go. Feel the silence.

One advantage of the audiotape over the videotape is that your focus won't be glued on the television but can be directed inward instead. Only your hearing will guide you, so although figuring out how to do a posture may be more difficult, many simpler postures, and especially breathing and meditation work, are perfect for the audiotape medium.

Whichever method is most helpful to you is the one you should pursue. Don't worry about what anyone else does. This is *your* yoga. A visit to your local library, video store, or bookstore will probably reveal a wealth of available videos and audiotapes you can borrow, rent, or buy. Try the library and the video store first. That way, you can sample a variety of yoga teachers and programs without committing. Once you've found a few you like, consider buying the tapes for your personal collection. Then, whenever the desire strikes (2:00 A.M. on a Tuesday, 11:00 P.M. on a Friday), you can do yoga!

Wise Yogi Tells Us

No matter how different we are from each other, we all have one very important and il-lustrious quality in common: We're all human! Keep in mind these six universal laws for being human:

➤ You will be given a body.

➤ You will be taught lessons.

➤ There are no mistakes in life, only lessons.

➤ If a lesson is not learned, it gets repeated.

➤ The more often a lesson is repeated, the harder it gets.

➤ You know you've learned your lesson when your actions change.

Yoga from Books

We hope you don't have the impression that you *can't* learn yoga from a book. For some, it's the only way! Remember *svadhyaya*, the *niyama* that encourages self-inquiry? Reading books on yoga and practicing from a book are part of this observance, which helps you understand yourself. Many excellent books on yoga exist, illustrating thousands of postures, breathing techniques, and meditation techniques. Books allow you to learn a broader spectrum of information than a teacher alone will probably be able to convey. Plus, you can go to the library and come home with 10 or 12 books on yoga—much easier than sampling 10 or 12 teachers!

Books cover yoga in a variety of ways—from an array of suggested workouts to the history of yoga to essays on spirituality to suggestions for daily yoga-friendly living. It's important to spend time reading, studying, and filling your mind with the types of ideas and concepts that inspire you. If you study a posture on the written level, your mind will understand it in a different way, and your body may even find it easier to follow. We can't always be movin' and shakin'!

If you thrive on reading, read to your heart's content—but don't *just* read. You also need to *act*. Get up and try what the book suggests. Following the postures from a picture and some text might be challenging at first, but once you find the posture, it will feel right, and pretty soon, you'll have your sequence of poses memorized.

But don't stop there! The more you learn about yoga, the wiser you'll be. Find books with more *asanas* you haven't tried yet. Check out the *Bhagavad Gita* (that classic Indian epic about *Krishna,* Prince Arjuna, and the meaning of life). Find a teacher whose views make sense to you, and read everything you can by and about him or her. You may find that as your life changes, your yoga goals and interests change and grow. Just go back to the library or the bookstore and find another book more in keeping with your developing state of mind. And always maintain a balance between reading and doing, doing and reading. Mind, body. Body, mind.

What better first book than the one you have in your hands? We hope this book is piquing your interest and that you have begun your yoga journey with us. After you've mastered this book, you won't feel like a "complete idiot" about yoga (even though you never *were,* as we explained in Chapter 1, "Why Practice Yoga?"). You'll be able to progress in your yoga practice with confidence and aplomb.

Yoga on the Net

For all you computer-heads and Internet lovers out there, despair not! The Internet is brimming with great yoga resources, from class information to "postures of the week" to peer support to spiritual guidance and inspiration. Of course, you always want to be careful when it comes to the people you talk to and where you send your money—use your common sense, then start surfing for yoga sites! Keep in mind that these Web sites do frequently change, as do their addresses. Here are a few to check out:

➤ **YOYOGA! with Joan** is Joan's (yes, the Joan co-authoring these very words!) marvelous yoga Web site with *asanas* of the week, yoga tips, and other wonderful wisdom, including the ever-popular "Yo Joan!" forum for all your yoga questions. Look up Joan at www.yoyoga.com.

➤ **Temple of Kriya Yoga Chicago,** where Joan studied, has a great Web site with plenty of resources and links. Check it out at www.yogakriya.org/.

➤ **The Yoga Anand Ashram** site contains lots of great poses and meditation information with pictures and clear explanations. It covers many aspects of yoga, and the site is user-friendly: www.santosha.com/.

➤ *Yoga Voices* is a printed monthly newsletter's online version, self-described as "dedicated to co-creating a healing community aligned with spirit, aligned with the resonation of unity and unconditional acceptance of all paths and all voices." The site includes an *asana* of the month and even poetry. Look it up at www.yogavoices.com.

➤ The *Yoga Journal* is probably the most famous yoga magazine and well worth the read. Browse through it at www.yogajournal.com.

➤ *Yoga International* is another excellent and popular yoga magazine. Check out highlights of current issues and back issues at www.earthchannel.com/ yogaintl/index.htm.

➤ **Yoga Site** is an "eclectic collection of yoga connections" and is full of yoga information, from philosophy to finding a teacher in your area. Great reading: www.yogasite.com.

➤ **YogaChicago** is a bi-monthly resource guide to yoga activities in the Chicago area and elsewhere: www.yogachicago.com/.

➤ **The Spirituality/Yoga/Hinduism** home page has beauty and brains—beautiful art, great graphics, and lots of information. Check it out at www.geocities.com/RodeoDrive/1415/index.html.

➤ **The Self-Realization Fellowship** is a worldwide religious organization dedicated to carrying on the spiritual and humanitarian work of Paramahansa Yogananda. Check it out at www.yogananda-srf.org/aboutsrf/index.html.

➤ **The Sivananda Yoga "OM"** page is the homepage of the International Sivananda Yoga Vedanta Center, a nonprofit organization founded by *Swami* Vishnu-devananda to spread the teachings of Yoga and Vedanta worldwide. Find them at www.sivananda.org/.

➤ **Himalayan International Institute of Yoga and Philosophy** combines Eastern wisdom and Western knowledge. The institute offers a wide variety of seminars and programs: www.himalayaninstitute.org.

A Yoga Minute

The world is full of wise *yogis*—even celebrities! These celebrities have all practiced yoga: Helen Hunt, Gwyneth Paltrow, Woody Harrelson, Jane Fonda, Oprah Winfrey, Madonna, Karen Allen, Sting, Quincy Jones, Ali McGraw, Ruth Buzzi, Tom Smothers, Carol Lynley, Justine Bateman, Jeff Bridges, John Saxon, Maud Adams, Herbie Hancock, Sarah Miles, and Dixie Carter.

Passage to India

Maybe you're serious about yoga—and we mean *really* serious. If you have the time, the resources, and the desire, you might consider actually venturing across the ocean and visiting yoga's homeland: India. After all, if you want to learn from the masters, shouldn't you go where the masters live?

Well, not necessarily. So many wonderful yoga masters have come to the United States to live and teach that you needn't traverse the ocean to meet or study with them. And yoga has been in the West for so long that many excellent teachers have been born and bred right here among us!

A trip to India may be more valuable for you if you are interested in exploring yoga's historical context, or if you are simply fascinated with the culture. Of course, India today is far more Westernized than it used to be, and it may not be what you expect. On the other hand, maybe it will meet your every expectation. If you're a traveler at heart and feel your own personal journey would be richly enhanced by the trip, go ahead!

But hold on—hang up the phone, don't call your travel agent just yet. If a trip to India interests you, you'll get the most from it if you spend a good deal of time and effort learning everything possible about yoga right where you are. Once you've learned what your own country can teach you, you'll have the knowledge, skill, and connections to reap the benefits of a trip to yoga's homeland. Check out the India Travel Promotion Network Web site at travel.indiamart.com/ or Lonely Planet's Destination India page at www.lonelyplanet.com/dest/ind/ind.htm.

And if the idea of a trip to India doesn't appeal to you? Of course that's fine! You can learn all you need to know right where you are. Wonderful, competent, and qualified yoga teachers exist in virtually every city, and you can practice yoga just as well in your own living room as you can on another continent (probably better!).

The Least You Need to Know

➤ Yoga is best learned from a good teacher in a class environment.

➤ Finding a teacher who is right for your personality is important for successful yoga practice.

➤ You can also learn yoga at home through books, video and audio cassettes, and the Internet.

➤ Going to India can be a rich, rewarding cultural experience, but you don't need to go there to do yoga.

Chapter 10

How to Practice Yoga

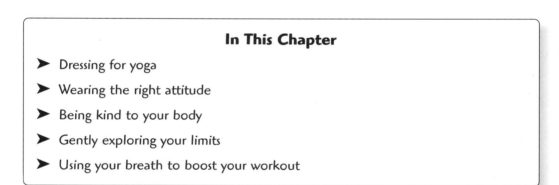

In This Chapter

➤ Dressing for yoga

➤ Wearing the right attitude

➤ Being kind to your body

➤ Gently exploring your limits

➤ Using your breath to boost your workout

Knowing how to practice yoga involves more than knowing how to do the postures. You won't be able to relax very easily in scratchy, stiff clothing that doesn't allow you to move freely. Likewise, the attitude you "wear" can hinder your practice. Learning to suspend your doubts, worries, and fears during your yoga practice is important for progress in your yoga journey. So is understanding when you are pushing yourself too hard, listening to your body to determine what it needs and what it doesn't need, and being prepared for deep breathing by knowing a few basic principles.

Loose Clothing and an Open Mind

You can't practice yoga well unless you're comfortable. The right clothing is important, because if you can't move easily, if your clothes are in the way, or if you are in any way unnecessarily distracted (say by a tight waist or stiff fabric), you won't be able to concentrate fully on your yoga postures.

There isn't any set yoga "uniform," but consider these points when deciding what to wear for your workout:

➤ Your clothes should be loose and flexible but not baggy. Tight clothes are restricting, and baggy clothes can get in the way of your movements. T-shirts and shorts or leggings, tank tops and biking shorts, or a not-too-baggy sweatsuit are ideal.

➤ Dress for the temperature. If the weather is cold, choose long sleeves and comfortable pants that don't restrict your movement (sweatpants or leggings are both good choices). Remember to keep a blanket nearby in case you get chilly.

➤ Your clothing shouldn't bind anywhere. If the feel of your clothes is very noticeable around your waist or at your ankles or wrists, they are probably too tight. Also, binding clothes will restrict the flow of energy through your body.

➤ You should be able to distinguish the basic shape of your body. Your teacher will need to see how you are holding the postures to make sure you are doing them correctly. If you are doing yoga on your own, relatively form-fitting clothing will allow you to check your form and alignment in a mirror without trying to imagine your form in a pose under that oversized T-shirt and those baggy pants.

➤ Yoga is best performed in bare feet. The more you practice yoga, the more sensitive and in tune with your environment you'll become, and that includes your feet!

➤ Don't forget to remove all metal jewelry before you practice, especially necklaces and bracelets. Yoga is about freeing the flow of energy in your body, and that energy could be disrupted by metal.

➤ Avoid wearing perfume, strongly scented deodorant, or cologne during your yoga practice. It can be unpleasant to others in your yoga class, especially during *pranayama* (breathwork).

➤ And what's the most important thing to wear? An open mind! The most perfect yoga outfit won't do you any good if you aren't mentally prepared. Before every yoga practice, take a few moments of quiet to prepare for your workout.

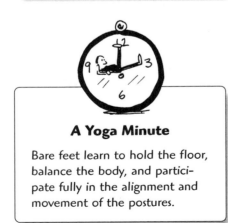

Wise Yogi Tells Us

If you have long hair, don't forget to tie it back before your yoga practice. There's nothing more frustrating than finally achieving a headstand after months of practice, only to get your hands tangled in your hair!

A Yoga Minute

Bare feet learn to hold the floor, balance the body, and participate fully in the alignment and movement of the postures.

Think about what you are about to do and what you want to accomplish. If you're just getting started, even if you aren't completely convinced yoga can do everything people say it can, willingly suspend your disbelief, just for a little while. An open mind means a body open to new movements and achievements. You may surprise yourself at what you can accomplish when you aren't wasting your energy doubting yourself and your workout.

Are You Kidding? My Body Won't Do That ...

Now that you're properly attired, you *look* like a *yogi*—but do you *feel* like a *yogi?* Maybe you're reluctant to begin that very first practice, because you know you aren't flexible or you're convinced you won't be able to achieve any of the postures you've heard about or seen.

The problem with an attitude of doubt is that it not only undermines your self-confidence, but it implies that you see yoga as a competition. We've said it before, but we can't emphasize enough how important this concept is, especially for competitive and goal-oriented people: Yoga is not a competitive sport! If you can't do the lotus position today, that doesn't matter one iota. Eventually, with regular practice, it will come. And even if it doesn't, it's still not a reflection on your ability as a *yogi.* You are much more than your body, and much more than the poses your body can achieve.

If you have a hard time relinquishing your competitive nature, try addressing your inner thoughts with these responses:

Your thought: *I'm much more flexible than that poor guy next to me!*

Your response to yourself: *My body is responding well today.*

Your thought: *I'll never be able to do a headstand!*

Your response to yourself: *I'll master this shoulderstand any day now, as long as I keep practicing. Maybe then I'll think about trying to learn the headstand.*

Your thought: *I think the teacher likes me best.*

Your response to yourself: *I've really found a teacher who understands me and my yoga needs.*

Your thought: *At this rate, I'll never be as flexible as that girl in the front.*

Your response to yourself: *That girl in front does that posture well. I'll try to visualize how it would feel to hold the posture that way, and maybe my body will understand the posture better.*

Your thought: *I look really hot in this new workout gear* or *I look really hot in this muscle shirt and bicycle shorts,* followed by *I wonder if there will be any cute guys/girls in the class.*

113

Your response to yourself: *I feel really good in these clothes. I think they will be great for yoga.* (What do you think your yoga class is, anyway—a singles' bar?)

Each posture you try should be a movement you're able to perform. Accept your current level of fitness and respect it. Also accept how you feel from day to day. You may be able to do postures one week that you suddenly are unable to achieve the next week. So many factors besides how "in shape" you are determine your ability to achieve a pose. Your mood, your stress level, the time of day, how well you have warmed up, your current feelings about yourself, the natural ebb and flow of your energy level—all these conditions will affect your workout. Each day, find your own movement and level.

Then start at that level, progressing as your body allows. Some days you may move ahead noticeably in your flexibility or strength. On other days, you may feel as if you have regressed. That's natural, and the regression will soon correct itself, so don't let it worry you. A good teacher can help you determine how fast you can advance, but you can also listen to your body, because it will tell you, too—as long as it isn't being overruled by your ego.

Remember that yoga is about toning down the ego. Your ego is what tells you to try to outdo the girl next to you or to match the picture in the book precisely. Your ego encourages you to try postures that are beyond your current fitness level, to hold postures too long, or to try the most difficult version of a posture first.

Wise Yogi Tells Us

Your ego lets seemingly nonchalant comments slip out of your mouth, such as "I could do the lotus pose the first time I tried," or "You found the plow position difficult? That's strange," or even, "I can't believe you could stand on one foot for so much longer than I could!" Let all that go. It doesn't help you. It only holds you back.

When your ego acts up ("How come I don't look like that when I do the shoulderstand?"), gently steer your mind in another direction. Remind yourself that this is your journey, and your progress is all that matters. The yoga road has no maximum or minimum speed limit!

No Pain, Supreme Gain

If you've ever participated in any team athletics, whether elementary school kickball or professional basketball, you've probably been told by some coach or teacher somewhere along the line that if it doesn't hurt (or isn't, at the very least, mildly unpleasant), you just aren't working hard enough.

The interesting thing about yoga, and one of its distinctly non-Western qualities, is that it allows you to work incredibly hard without ever feeling pain, discomfort, or even displeasure of any kind. Yoga should be innately enjoyable because …

➤ It doesn't hurt. Causing yourself pain would be to ignore the observance of *ahimsa* (nonviolence).

➤ It boosts *all* of you. A successful yoga workout increases self-esteem, along with fitness and awareness.

➤ It purifies your body, mind, and soul. Being clean feels good!

➤ Even at its most serious, yoga is just plain fun!

Yoga should never cause you pain. Pain means violence and possibly injury. Violence and injury mean a setback. Better to move slowly and steadily forward than to jump ahead in leaps and bounds, then fall back bedridden for a month. You'll gain so much more strength, flexibility, sensitivity, and awareness if you are so attuned to your body that you push it to its limit, but never far enough to hurt anything. Respect your body, don't abuse it—it's an integral part of you, after all.

Of course, none of us is perfect, and in any physical activity, occasionally we all overdo it, especially when we're trying to outdo someone (even ourselves!). We know you're trying to listen to your body and not be competitive. But just in case, watch out for these signs that you may have injured yourself:

➤ Severe back pain and muscle spasms could be a sign of a back sprain, often caused by a sudden bending of the spine that tears ligaments.

➤ Immediate, acute shoulder pain that gets worse over the course of a few hours may be caused by a tear in the tendons and/or muscles around the shoulder joint. A severe tear may inhibit movement and can be caused by a minor fall on an outstretched hand.

➤ Pain in the knee and an inability to straighten the knee, followed by swelling that lasts for two weeks or more, may be due to torn cartilage. This can happen when a bent knee is twisted.

➤ Foot pain from standing for excessive amounts of time or overusing the foot can result in a strain or sprain.

➤ Dizziness can be a sign of low or high blood pressure or blood sugar levels. If you become dizzy, sit down immediately. Check this condition with your doctor.

➤ Headaches can have numerous sources. One reason people get headaches is because of insufficient oxygen. *Pranayama* to the rescue! Breathing exercises may help your headaches, and the stress-reducing aspects of yoga can also be helpful for this common problem.

A Yoga Minute

Surveys of industrialized nations show that more than 75 percent of the population over 45 years of age suffers from lower back pain.

Ouch!

If you happen to overdo it during your yoga workout and find yourself in serious pain, do yourself a favor and *go to your healthcare provider immediately!* Ignoring the pain won't make it go away and, in some cases, could result in a serious or chronic health problem. Just do it.

Of course, the best way to handle an injury is to prevent it. Stay alert to your body. Communicate with your muscles and joints. Be kind to them. Remember *ahimsa* (nonviolence)!

Finding the Edge vs. Feeling the Burn

"But if yoga is so easy on your body, how are you supposed to get anywhere?" you may wonder. Hey, we never said yoga was easy! Yoga isn't always easy. Sometimes it's downright difficult. Just because you aren't committing violence to your body doesn't mean a yoga workout is akin to a day of sunbathing at the beach. On the contrary: Yoga can be tough and intensely challenging.

The difference between yoga and other types of exercise is that the challenge and the progression are deeply internal and subtle. Perhaps you've been trying to accomplish a pose in which you bend forward and touch your head to your knees. The first time you try it, you don't even come close. You can barely bend forward without your back causing you pain, so bend your knees and slowly work at bringing the head and upper body down. Slowly build so that your back strengthens and you can straighten your knees. Lean into your farthest point in the stretch and hold it. Remember to keep breathing, letting your breath travel through your body and into the pose. Holding the pose won't hurt (not exactly), but you'll definitely feel something. Your muscles may shake a bit, and that's okay, as long as you aren't forcing the issue. You may even break a sweat. You're feeling the "edge" of your flexibility as well as an edge of your awareness. Your muscles are waking up and saying, "Hey! What is it you want us to do? This is weird, but okay, we'll give it a try." Your mind is waking up, too, and taking notice.

The next time you try this pose, you get a little closer—maybe three or four inches from your knees. The farthest point of the stretch is now a little farther than it was before. You stretch to this point and hold it. Now your muscles have become accustomed to a new "normal" level of flexibility. You find the new edge and test it—not to the point of pain, but just to see where it now lies. Your muscles feel it, and so does your mind.

A few weeks, or months, or maybe a lifetime later (how long it takes isn't important, because it's not a competition), you lean into the stretch and … wow! There it is! Suddenly your head is resting quite easily on your knees. You've stretched your boundaries and pushed your edge to a new level. At this point, you may simply feel triumphant, but you may also feel an awakening to a new level of yourself. No longer simply proud of your achievement, you're now aware of yourself in a new way.

Therein lies yoga's power—the physical process breaking into the mental process and lifting the whole of you to higher and higher states of awareness.

Keep in mind that every posture contains an "edge" or a point past which—for today, at least—you can't quite go. This is the point around which you want to linger, because it's the source of yoga's power. You'll soon see how productive it is to recognize an edge but not let it define you.

Don't Forget to Breathe

And once again, we remind you of your ever-present breath. Although breathing exercises are performed separately from the postures, breathing is also important during the postures. Of course, you have to breathe while exercising, but becoming aware of your breath, even breathing in a specific way according to the posture you are holding, will enhance your practice and help your body work better.

Here are a few breath-savvy concepts to keep in mind while practicing your *asanas:*

➤ Inhalation most often occurs when your chest opens, your limbs extend outward or upward, and your head is up.

➤ Exhalation most often occurs when your chest contracts inward, your limbs move close to your body, your head is down, and your body curls into itself.

➤ Retaining the breath after an inhalation helps stabilize and energize the chest area.

➤ Retaining the breath after an exhalation helps stabilize and energize the abdominal area, and releases toxins from the body.

➤ Forward-bending poses are conducive to exhalation, then retention.

➤ Backbending poses are conducive to inhalation, then retention.

Wise Yogi Tells Us

Your breath has four modes:

➤ Inhalation

➤ Exhalation

➤ Retained breath after inhalation

➤ Retained breath after exhalation

Learning how to use each mode when it is most beneficial will greatly enhance your practice.

Breathing deeply and well during exercise keeps a steady supply of oxygen in the blood so muscles can work at their peak. Breathing keeps the mind calm and focused, which will further enhance your workout. And since the breath is the vehicle by which *prana,* the universal life force, enters the body, you'll certainly want to breathe

117

deeply during your workout. *Prana* is the energy that keeps you vibrant and animated. It's the key to a great workout, so get as much into you as possible! Breathe! Breathe! Breathe!

Ouch!

If you become out of breath or fatigued during your workout, stop! Yoga isn't circuit training, marathon running, or nonstop anything. Rest is encouraged within a workout—as a transition from one type of posture to another, as a chance to feel the aftereffects of a posture, and to maintain awareness. Bodies aren't meant to be exhausted but to be gently and lovingly improved and maintained.

The Least You Need to Know

➤ Wear comfortable clothing during yoga.

➤ Don't be competitive.

➤ Don't force any posture until it hurts, but keep exploring your limits.

➤ If you have any lingering pain, consult a doctor immediately; don't wait for it to become chronic.

➤ Breathe deeply and often!

Chapter 11

When to Practice Yoga

In This Chapter

➤ Making a schedule

➤ Sticking with it

➤ Squeezing yoga into your busy day

➤ Revitalizing with yoga throughout the day

Time, time, time ... never enough of it, and it just keeps on passing us by. During the course of our busy lives, it's easy to become overwhelmed by the demands on our time. Family, friends, work, school, home ... all require their share. The furnace needs to be repaired, the dishes are dirty, the kids need to be picked up from soccer practice or ballet or the baby-sitters. You can't neglect time with your spouse, you have to finish the inventory at work, the baby needs some serious cuddling ... and has anyone walked the dog lately?

Or maybe you're a student. You have five papers due in the next month. Calculus has completely eluded you. Seven chemistry problems are due tomorrow, and you're also supposed to have finished *War and Peace* by last week. Your roommate won't turn down the music, the library is closed because of a flood, and it's just starting to thunder, so studying outside isn't an option. You hear a rumor that your history teacher is planning a pop quiz for tomorrow.

And we're suggesting you add some time for yoga?

Yep. And you'll be glad we suggested it, too. You do have time for yoga, even if it doesn't seem like you could possibly track down one spare second. All it takes is a little organization and some creative thinking.

Time to get organized! All great accomplishments start with some type of plan. An effective yoga practice has a plan involving two important aspects:

➤ How often will you practice each week?

➤ What will you do during the course of each practice?

Ouch!

Always practice yoga on an empty stomach. Just before breakfast or dinner is ideal. Digestion will interfere with what yoga is trying to accomplish in your body, and a full stomach will make exercise uncomfortable. Your whole body, including your internal organs, should be focused on your practice, not on processing that spaghetti dinner!

The first question depends a lot on your schedule, your motivation, and your desire. Ideally, yoga should be practiced three to six times per week. If you take a class once a week, that counts as a practice. Then practice on your own using the routine you and your teacher have crafted for you. Or, if you are on your own, set up a specific schedule of yoga days. A regular schedule is the best way to reap yoga's benefits. Yes, even just once a week counts as a regular schedule (but you may soon find that once a week won't be enough, and you'll find more time, and more ...).

When planning your weekly yoga schedule, remember that even though yoga isn't harsh on your body, you should still give yourself at least one day every week to rest. Rest is crucial for yoga. The time spent in *asanas* (postures) is balanced by the time spent resting, and it is this rest time when the body heals and replenishes its resources. Or, rest every other day. Survey the following list of suggested yoga schedules, and choose one that fits your life, or modify one to suit you:

❑ Monday, Wednesday, and Friday: Yoga 20 minutes before work.

Tuesday, Thursday, and the weekend: Rest.

❑ Monday through Friday: Yoga for 30 minutes right after work.

Weekend: Rest.

❑ Tuesday and Thursday: Yoga for 15 minutes first thing in the morning (energizing poses) and 15 minutes before bed (relaxing poses).

Weekend: Yoga for 30 minutes in the afternoon.

Monday, Wednesday, and Friday: Rest.

❑ Saturday and Sunday: Yoga for 60 minutes.

Monday through Friday: Rest.

❑ Saturday: Yoga for 60 minutes.

Sunday through Friday: Rest.

Once you have a schedule, keep it in your head, write it down, post it on the refriger-
ator … whatever it takes. Then follow your schedule! Remember *tapas,* the *niyama*
about self-discipline? Here's a great chance to use it. You'll feel great about yourself if
you faithfully stick to your yoga schedule.

Now what about the schedule for your routine itself? Your teacher can help you craft
the perfect yoga practice for you, taking into consideration any special needs you
have or problems you'd like yoga to address (bad knees, allergies, back pain, frazzled
nerves). Or refer to Appendix A, "Yoga Sessions for the Time You Have," for various
suggested routines after reading Chapter 12, "Crafting Your Personalized Yoga
Practice," to more clearly define your own purpose.

Don't forget that every yoga practice should include the following:

➤ **A warm-up.** It's important to get your muscles warm and activated before you start
stretching them. Warm-ups help prevent injury and make a wonderful transition from
daily life to yoga mode. A short walk in the
fresh air makes a great warm-up, because it
sends blood to all your muscles and gets
those joints moving. (The quality of your
walk is more important than the length; use
the time to prepare your body and mind.)
You can get a similar effect simply by massag-
ing your legs, feet, arms, and hands. Work
those muscles and joints to get them ready
for action. If you're lucky enough to know a
massage therapist, a professional massage before (or after!) yoga practice can be therapeutic. You might also try a warm shower or
bath, or a heating pad on stiff areas, to warm
your muscles before your workout.

Wise Yogi Tells Us

The most spiritual time of day
and the most ideal for practicing
yoga is just before sunrise (about
5:30 A.M.). If you make it a habit
to practice yoga before sunrise,
then relax with a cup of herbal
tea to watch the dawn, you'll
find a new sense of peace per-
vading your days. And to think
you've been sleeping through all
that beauty!

➤ **A balanced set of poses.** Postures that bend or twist to one side should be balanced with postures that bend or twist to the other side. Forward bends balance
backbends. Right-side-up poses balance inverted poses. Poses that stretch and
expand are balanced by poses that curl and contract. Energizing poses balance
relaxing poses. You get the idea.

➤ **Every yoga workout should conclude with the final relaxation, or corpse
posture.** In this pose, mighty healing takes place … for your body and mind.
Don't neglect this pose because you think you don't have time to just lie there.
It's probably the most important of all the postures. (See Chapter 19, "Dead to
the World.")

121

➤ *Pranayama,* **or breathing exercises.** Remember those breathing techniques from Chapter 7, "Can You Breathe?" After you practice your *asanas,* set aside a short time for the practice of a breathing technique or two. Replenish your body's *prana,* or life force!

➤ *Dhyana,* **or meditation.** You might not be ready to include meditation in your workout. If that's the case, that's fine. Diligently practice your *asanas* and *pranayama,* and you may find that meditation soon becomes a more compelling prospect. Or, if you would like to try it but are short on time, you might consider meditating at a different time of day. Whenever you meditate (after your *asanas* and *pranayama* or during separate sessions), remember that meditation is part of yoga, too, and will have a direct benefit on your workout. (Your workout will have a direct benefit on your meditation efforts, as well.)

Wise Yogi Tells Us

If you're feeling depressed or even just a little blue, which should you do—meditation or postures? If you guessed postures, you're right! The action of the postures is designed to move impurities and negativity out of the body. Meditation, on the other hand, involves stillness and concentration. If you are filled with negative feelings, meditation could actually concentrate them and make you feel worse. Meditation is best practiced in a positive frame of mind.

Here's a rhyme to help you remember:

If you're down, move around. Feeling great? Meditate!

Sticking with It

To really get the most out of yoga, a commitment is in order. Although occasional yoga is better than no yoga, life changes and dramatic benefits will come more quickly and easily if you practice yoga regularly, whether that means a few times a week or a few times a day. Commitment-phobic, are you? Don't be! This is a relationship with yourself, so even though you might discover some surprises (what relationship doesn't have a few of those?), this commitment is well worth the effort you put into it.

A Yoga Minute

Whatever questions or issues seem personally relevant or important to you should be the subject of your journal entries. Keeping written track of your practice in this way will not only encourage you to practice regularly, but will also serve as a valuable and interesting record for the more advanced *yogi* you will be in the future. Someday it may be fun and enlightening to see how far you've come and what path you took.

Still, even for the most well-intentioned, cultivating a new habit can be difficult at first. If you're having trouble sticking to your yoga schedule, try the following strategies. One of them may be just the inspiration you need.

➤ **Let's make a deal.** First yoga, *then* breakfast. No yoga, no food. Or first yoga, then a long, hot bubble bath. No yoga, no bath. Whatever deal you make with yourself, be firm. At first, breakfast, a bubble bath, or whatever your deal involves will seem like a reward, but before long, yoga will become its own reward and you won't need to make any more deals—unless they involve using your yoga practice as the reward! (If I clean the whole kitchen, then I get to practice yoga for 30 whole minutes!)

➤ **It's a family affair.** Get your partner or kids involved! When you don't feel like practicing, someone else in the family probably will, and that can be enough of a motivation. (Who could deny a preschooler begging to "play" yoga?) Conversely, when your partner or kids are feeling less than motivated, you may be the one to encourage them. (See Chapter 25, "Yoga for the Whole Family.")

➤ **Associate yoga with another pleasurable activity, then always link them.** To use a previous example, every time you get up early to do yoga, you also get to relax with a cup of tea and watch the sunrise. Or whenever you do yoga, your family knows they can't bother you for an entire 30 minutes, or however long you can convince them to do without you. Maybe you can even work up to a whole, glorious hour! Yoga will mean peace, relaxation—time for you, and you alone.

➤ **Keep a yoga journal.** Every day that you practice yoga, take a few moments in the morning or evening (or whenever you have time) to write down how long you practiced, what time of day it was, exactly what you did, and then, most

123

important, how you feel about it. Did you make progress today? Did you feel like you experienced a setback? How do you feel now? Are you still carrying the feeling of your practice, or is it gone? How is your stress level? Don't feel you have to address all or even any of these questions—they are just suggestions.

➤ **Put yoga on your to-do list.** Put it right alongside all your other important daily duties, then check it off when you have finished. Subconsciously, you may not be giving yoga a high priority, and that's why it's so easy to forget or put off. Consciously placing yoga high on your list, equal to (if not higher than) such important tasks as getting the car fixed, turning in that report to your boss, or buying the groceries for your big dinner party, may be the motivation you need to accomplish your yoga practice every time it's scheduled.

Maybe another strategy will work better for you, but have a strategy! Commitments require a plan, but ideas without a plan rarely amount to anything. Take your yoga seriously, commit, exercise a little self-discipline, or simply allow yoga to be so fun and refreshing that you wouldn't possibly skip a workout! Soon you'll have no trouble making yoga a natural part of your life.

Ouch!

Your body reacts differently to stress than to relaxation. Compare these physiological responses:

Stress

➤ Heart rate increases.

➤ Muscle tension increases.

➤ Breathing rate increases.

➤ Blood pressure increases.

➤ Blood-clotting time decreases.

Relaxation

➤ Heart rate decreases.

➤ Muscle tension decreases.

➤ Breathing rate decreases.

➤ Blood pressure decreases.

➤ Blood-clotting time increases.

Yoga Bytes at Home, School, and Work

If you're an extremely busy person, as most of us seem to be these days, you may find it difficult to find time for yoga. Perhaps you think your day is so densely packed with activity that yoga will never fit. Don't despair! The great thing about yoga is that you get big results even when you spend just a little time each day.

Three 10-minute (or even 5-minute or 3-minute) slots for postures, the first for warmups, the second for more strenuous postures, and the third for relaxation postures, are all you need to start practicing yoga, and you can spread them throughout the day if necessary. You may find that the increased energy you gain magically adds time to your day for even more practice!

You can even slip tiny little "yoga bytes" into your day to keep you focused and feeling great. Try squeezing in yoga during the following "free times" at home, school, and the office.

Yoga on the Home Front

Here are some yoga bytes to try at home:

➤ Get up 10 minutes before the rest of the family to practice. Morning is a great time to practice the cat pose. Get down on your hands and knees, then arch your back up as high as you can while lowering your head. Imagine you are a cat stretching after a long nap. Then relax your back and bring your head up. Do this a few times, breathing with the movements. This exercise keeps your spine limber and gets you ready to pounce on the new day!

➤ Practice right after your shower, before getting dressed. Try the lightning bolt pose to get your energy soaring. (See Chapter 13, "What Do You Stand For?")

➤ Practice the mountain pose while waiting for the pasta to boil (see Chapter 13). Watch the bubbles slowly building and rising to the surface. What powerful forces are heat and energy! Reflect on how to choose to use the "bubbles" that inevitably build up inside you.

➤ Practice while waiting for the laundry to dry. Stand behind a chair. Place your hands on the chair's back. Take a large step back. While continuing to hold onto the chair, straighten your arms out and bend forward. Now lift one leg straight out behind you. Balance. This pose strengthens the legs and stretches the spine.

➤ Practice deep breathing while running your bath water. (See Chapter 7.)

➤ Practice your regular yoga routine while the rest of the family is watching television. (Eventually they may decide what you are doing is more interesting and join you!)

➤ Practice with the kids for a family-bonding yoga session. Kids usually love yoga, especially moving like different animals. Try the cat pose (described earlier in this list). Everyone purrrr like a cat! Then try the tree pose (see Chapter 13). Ask your kids what it's like to be a tree. Be a family of trees in different kinds of weather—a gentle breeze, a thrashing thunderstorm, a perfectly still day. Are your trees sturdy and strong, or young and flexible? Does the wind barely stir them, lash them all around, or knock them right down?

➤ Practice just before you go to sleep, but stick to relaxation postures such as the lotus pose (see Chapter 17, "Are You Sitting Down?"), the child's pose (see Chapter 18, "Take the Forward Path"), or *shavasana*, the corpse pose (see Chapter 19). Otherwise, you may be too energized for slumber.

Know Your Sanskrit

Shavasana, also known as the corpse pose (*shava* means "corpse"), is perhaps the most important of all the yoga *asanas* and involves total relaxation while lying, "corpse-like," on the ground. *Shavasana* is a surprisingly challenging pose. It isn't easy to lie still!

School Days

Yoga bytes for the stressed-out student:

➤ Are you nervous about a test you are taking? Breathe! Increase your exhalation so it's longer than your inhalation. Do this a few times. Come back to the test. This type of breathwork releases toxins from your body and centers your mind.

➤ Feeling a lot of tension in your back? Sit up straight. Keep both knees and feet together and facing forward. Twist your upper body. Bring one arm around the back of your chair. Do not overtwist your neck. Look behind you. This movement improves circulation to the spine and brain. It also improves flexibility and eyesight.

➤ As you walk across campus from class to class in the fresh air, take a moment to focus on your surroundings. Breathe the fresh air. Feel the sun on your face, the wind in your hair. Instead of worrying about the test you just took, the quiz you are about to take, or the paper due tomorrow, let all your worries go—just for a minute!—and live wholly in the moment.

Yoga Makes Work Less Work!

Here are a few yoga bytes you might like to try at the office if your situation permits:

➤ **Practice on your coffee break instead of drinking coffee.** (Yoga is far more energizing, once you break that caffeine addiction!) Sit with your fingers wide apart on top of your knees. Inhale deeply. Open your mouth wide and stick out your tongue. Look up and exhale strongly. Repeat the process a few times (not in front of your boss!). This releases emotions, tensions in the face, and self-consciousness. It also helps to break a depression cycle.

➤ **Practice right before your lunch hour.**
While sitting, as you take a long inhale,
stretch one leg straight out in front of you
and hold it up parallel to the floor. Pull your
toes back toward your head. Hold for three
counts. Lower your leg as you slowly exhale.
Do each leg a few times. This improves your
hip joints and strengthens your legs so your
knees won't be as stiff when you stand.

➤ **At the end of a long work day, pause for a
moment to get centered and refocus before
you head home.** Stand up and stretch your
arms up over your head. Look up. Bend forward and touch the ground. Bend your knees
if you need to. You have just connected the
sun to the earth. After an accomplishment
like that, you're ready to head home.

Ouch!

Eyestrain can result from staring
at a computer all day. Try a yoga
fix: Keeping your head still, look
up as far as you can, focus on
something, and count to three.
Look down, focus, and count to
three. Repeat six or seven times,
focusing in different directions,
then close your eyes and rest.
When you open your eyes,
they'll feel remarkably refreshed.

Yoga Renewal

Depending on what time of day you practice yoga, you can experience different kinds
of renewal. We humans are deeply affected by the time of day. We all have a *circadian*
(daily) *rhythm,* or physiological rhythms associated with the 24-hour clock. Have you
noticed you have more energy in the morning, the late afternoon, or at night? Are
you a "morning person" or a "night person"? Are you usually hungrier at a certain
time of day, or sleepier, or happier, or more depressed? Probably, if you take the time
to notice, you'll be able to determine how your feelings, emotions, and energies
change throughout the day. So it only makes sense that morning yoga, afternoon
yoga, and evening yoga will all be a little different. And remember, yoga is *about*
rhythm and balance—of body, mind, and spirit. Our very lives move to the rhythm
of our heartbeat and our breath.

Although each person's rhythms are different, people have a few similar tendencies.
Keep these points in mind when deciding what time of day to practice yoga:

➤ Early morning yoga tends to be slower. Do not rush into postures. Gently and
steadily move through your workout.

➤ Late-morning to midday yoga will probably be more intense. The body is awake
now and ready to rock and roll (literally!). This is a perfect time for *vinyasa,* a
way to practice yoga that involves a steady flow of yoga postures.

➤ Afternoon yoga is centering. The body naturally takes a siesta in the mid-
afternoon, so a more intense workout may help you get through this time.

If you end your workout with *shavasana* (the corpse pose), you'll be ready for the rest of your day.

➤ Evening or late-night yoga is unwinding. Let the strain of a busy day float away. If your day was unusually stressful, an intense *Hatha Yoga* workout will help to release tensions before you go into a nice, long *shavasana*.

No matter when you practice, yoga will renew you. Yoga has many purposes—among them, to energize, heal, relax, realign, and inspire you. But all paths and purposes lead to renewal, or a new you, free from stress and preoccupation with the self.

The Least You Need to Know

➤ Establish a plan that works for you—how often you will practice yoga and what you will do in each practice. It doesn't take much time!

➤ When starting out, strategies such as getting the family involved or keeping a yoga journal can help you stick with your practice.

➤ You can easily fit in short yoga practices throughout your day.

➤ Yoga can help relieve tension at home, school, and work.

➤ Your yoga workout will differ depending on when you practice.

Chapter 12

Crafting Your Personalized Yoga Practice

> ### In This Chapter
>
> ➤ Defining your yoga purpose
>
> ➤ Knowing your own style improves your yoga practice
>
> ➤ A yoga essay test
>
> ➤ Learning from your answers
>
> ➤ Ground rules for yoga practice

Just as it's important to have a plan for your yoga practice, it's also important to have a purpose. If you don't really know *why* you want to practice yoga, you won't really know *how* to practice yoga. You're an individual, and you bring a unique mix of motivations, emotions, tendencies, biases, needs, wants, and traits to your practice. Being familiar with all of these will not only help you determine which postures will be best for you, but will also be a great help to your yoga commitment.

Define Your Purpose

What are you looking to gain from your yoga practice?

- ❏ I'm primarily looking for a good fitness program.
- ❏ I'm in need of stress reduction.
- ❏ I suffer from a physical condition that I believe yoga could alleviate.

❏ Eastern philosophy fascinates me.

❏ I want to increase my mind power.

❏ I like the idea of a holistic fitness program.

❏ I'm interested in yoga because I've seen how it has benefited others.

If you really aren't sure, take some time to relax and dig deep into your mind. Think about why you want to be a *yogi*. You'll get some ideas if you just give yourself time to ponder the question.

Wise Yogi Tells Us

When you start to analyze yourself, your motives, your intentions, and your personality, try to be as objective as possible. Don't judge yourself, just see yourself. Try to be like a mirror. A mirror doesn't say, "Hey, you look great today!" or "Whoa, you'd better not go out looking like that!" Your ego says those things. Be the mirror. Just reflect.

A Yoga Minute

Spell the word *guru* out loud: G-U-R-U. Yes, you are! Good for you!

Sense Your Style

Before you begin your yoga practice you'll also want to get in touch with who you are. What is it about you, the individual, that will make your yoga experience unique?

❏ I am naturally energetic.

❏ I am resistant to exercise.

❏ I am an optimist. I am a pessimist.

❏ I am most concerned with the physical me. The intellectual me. The emotional me.

❏ I am easily excited.

❏ I am the calm, relaxed type.

❏ I consider myself self-confident.

Even if you aren't sure about the answers to these questions, give them some thought, too. Take the time to get to know yourself. The point of this entire chapter, and especially of the following "test," is to get you in touch with who you are so yoga can do its job.

A Yoga Essay Test You Can't Fail

If you break out in a cold sweat at the thought of a test, think of this as a self-evaluation. No one else will read your answers (unless you show them to someone), so be as honest as you possibly can. Don't try to fool yourself. Your yoga journey will be better and more fulfilling if you really understand your goals, motivations, and desires.

For each question, write what first comes into your mind, and here's a new twist—keep on writing for a minute or two. Even if you feel you've answered the question in one sentence, continue on and write anything that occurs to you, but try to keep closely focused on the question. This exercise is called "freewriting," and you might be surprised at what leaps out of your subconscious mind and onto the page. We suggest that you use these self-evaluation exercises to begin your yoga journal. After you've been practicing yoga for a period of time, say six months, return to the self-evaluation and see if you'd still answer all the questions the same way.

Don't feel you have to hurry through this test. You don't even have to complete it in one session. But try to complete it before you dive into your yoga practice. Just as a doctor needs to understand all of a patient's symptoms before making a diagnosis, so you should fully understand your own physical, emotional, mental, and spiritual states before you start to improve them.

Remember the most important thing when completing this test: Don't censor yourself! Write what you really feel about each question. Seriously think about who you are and what you—not anyone else—think about the question. Don't even consider what you "should" think (whatever *that* means!). Just feel whatever it is you *do* think. Let it all hang out, and then we'll take a look at who we're dealing with: you!

Wise Yogi Tells Us

If you have a hard time analyzing your own personality, imagine you're someone else who's just met you. Try to look at yourself through the eyes of another person. What's your first impression of this new friend (you)?

Ouch!

Thinking negatively about yourself—negative self-talk—can become a habit. Breaking this nasty habit can be difficult, but it's possible. First, make an effort to notice when you feel negative. Second, consciously try to rephrase your negative thoughts into positive ones. Eventually you'll retrain your mind to accentuate the positive!

1. If I had to describe myself to someone who doesn't know me, I would say:

_____

2. I have an "outer me" I show to the world and an "inner me" that's more private. Here's how I'd describe the "inner me"—the qualities I have that people might not notice at first, or that I consider mine alone and not necessarily for sharing:

_____

3. (If you have anything even slightly negative in your answers to the first two questions, underline it.) Now: I could argue that the negative qualities I mentioned are also positive qualities when I look at them this way:

_____

4. My best friends would describe me as:

_____

5. When I'm confronted with someone who has different beliefs than mine, I feel:

_____

6. If I could give one of my personal qualities to everyone in the entire world in order to make it a better place, I'd give everyone my:

_____

7. The qualities in someone else that spark my admiration are:

_____

8. This is the way I feel about my chosen profession, especially in terms of how it reflects my personality and satisfies my needs and ambitions:

_____

9. If someone stole my parking space, would I be more likely to react physically (for example, jump out of the car and deck them), verbally (shout at them, swear profusely, or say something nasty about their appearance or intelligence), or emotionally (think to myself that the person is a jerk, imagine elaborate scenarios of revenge, or brood on the incident all day)? This is how I would be likely to act:

_____

10. I think the greatest thing about the world today is:

_____

11. I think some of the problems with the world today are:

_____

12. I think the greatest thing about me is:

_____

13. Here are my thoughts on the existence of a divine power:

_____

14. If I could change one thing about the world, it would be:

_____

15. If I could change one thing about myself, it would be:

_____

16. I bought this book because:

    _____

17. I think it will be important for my yoga teacher to have certain qualities, such as:

    _____

18. I hope to accomplish the following from my yoga practice (ranked in order of importance):

    a. _____

    b. _____

    c. _____

    d. _____

    e. _____

19. Since yoga is about more than touching your toes, if someone is in a difficult yoga pose, are they necessarily doing yoga? Explain some reasons why or why not.

    _____

20. Considering all of these questions, I can think of five reasons why yoga might benefit me personally:

    a. _____

    b. _____

    c. _____

    d. _____

    e. _____

Let's Get Personal

See, that wasn't so bad! We hope you even thought it was kind of fun! And now that you're finished, it's time to score your test. Here goes: You get an A+. It's true! You answered every single question correctly.

If you find that, when evaluating yourself, most of your answers are negative ones ("I'm selfish," "I have low self-esteem," "I don't have very many friends," etc.), nip that negative self-talk in the bud! Whenever you catch yourself forming a negative thought, restate it in the positive ("I am aware of my needs," "I often put others first," "I have a few really good friends").

This test has no wrong answers, but that doesn't diminish your accomplishment. You have undertaken a fairly intense self-evaluation, and what you have learned will only make your yoga practice more fulfilling and effective. Continue to think about your answers to these test questions as you go through your day. Consider it the beginning of a beautiful friendship with your higher self.

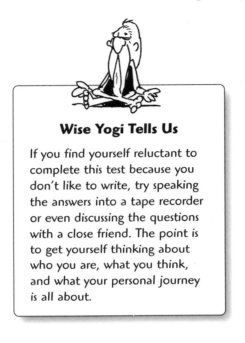

Wise Yogi Tells Us

If you find yourself reluctant to complete this test because you don't like to write, try speaking the answers into a tape recorder or even discussing the questions with a close friend. The point is to get yourself thinking about who you are, what you think, and what your personal journey is all about.

The first step is getting to know all of you—even the parts of you that you aren't so proud of. The next step is learning to be proud of the whole package. We hope you have a better idea of your own self-concept after taking this quiz, but even if you aren't completely pleased with what you discover, the most important thing you can do now is accept yourself. You are a unique individual, and you are human. You may think you're not perfect, and, or, that nobody is perfect. We could argue that, deep down, everyone is perfect.

But we are all moving through life, exploring who we are, where we are, and why we are. We're all working toward self-discovery at our own pace.

Take it easy on yourself. You're working at your own speed and learning as you go, like the rest of us. You are an amazing person, worthy of self-respect and self-love. In fact, you are miraculous. Feel good about who you are and where you are, and yoga will be a natural avenue of self-care.

Yoga Ground Rules

In the next chapter, we'll actually start learning different yoga postures, or *asanas*. But before we do, let's examine a few ground rules that apply to every posture. Actually, these are not rules so much as sound advice and helpful hints to encourage you to optimize your yoga practice and make the most of each moment.

First, let's look at some general rules for poses. Before you start posturing, keep these important yoga tips in mind:

➤ Hold each pose for three breaths (both inhalation and exhalation) to start, and gradually increase the time you hold each pose, as you're able to do so.

➤ Don't feel you have to look just like the picture! More important, find peace within each pose, and progress as your body allows you to.

➤ For each pose, make sure you have a counterpose to keep your body balanced. For example, bends to the right should be balanced with bends to the left, forward bends with backbends, contractions with expansions, and so on.

➤ Generally speaking, exhale as you go into forward bends and inhale as you go into backbends.

Posture Perfect

Good posture is essential to proper form in yoga. It also helps allow your body to achieve or maintain good health. It feels better, looks better, and *is* better for your body. Good posture also influences your feelings and thoughts. If you stand up straight and tall, you'll think more positive thoughts. It's true! Try it!

Good posture extends beyond the practice of your yoga postures. You spend a lot of your life standing—but do you stand well? The next time the fact that you're standing comes to mind, notice how you're doing it, whether you're in line at the grocery store, filling up at the gas station, or stir-frying vegetables at the stove.

Chances are, you'll notice that your posture is less than straight, tall, aligned, and balanced. Maybe you carry one shoulder higher or lower than the other. Maybe you shift your weight to one hip, or stoop forward, or lean your head to the left or right. Even if you're fairly balanced, you may not be standing as tall as you could be, and your muscles may not be in command over gravity or bad habits.

Posture is more important to your health than many people realize. Ask any chiropractor—if the body isn't aligned, the energy gets "clogged" in certain areas and doesn't flow freely. If part of you is energy deprived, you're out of balance, and the more out of balance you become, the greater your chances of succumbing to stress, depression, and disease. Good posture helps a body to heal itself, so help your body to be its best. Mountain pose, in the next chapter, can help you train your body to stand straight and tall.

A misaligned body can impede the flow of energy. It doesn't look good, but more important, it can keep your body from achieving optimal physical and emotional health.

135

Wise Yogi Tells Us

Here's an easy way to maintain good posture while standing: Pretend that you have a loop attached to the crown of your head, and a string tied to the loop. Imagine someone above you is pulling on the string. Feel how your entire spine and neck shift and stretch as the string pulls upward. That's what good posture feels like!

Ouch!

Don't get tense about the "warrior" idea. Some people hear the word and their muscles immediately tense up as if they're preparing for battle. Yet the most effective warriors stay calm, clear-headed, and in a position to move in any direction as the situation requires. You can achieve this readiness without debilitating tension by concentrating on internally lifting the center of your body.

Moving Mountains

You may be tempted to flip to the back of the book to look for the poses you think look more difficult or impressive. We urge you to stay right where you are! Standing poses, and mountain pose in particular, provide an important training ground for all the yoga *asanas*. If you don't know how to stand like a mountain, all your other poses will show it.

Let's consider the importance of standing poses. Standing poses develop and strengthen your legs, those all-important limbs and vehicles of motion. Standing poses also improve your balance, align your hips and spine, and maintain equilibrium throughout your body. Master the standing poses before you attempt to master the more complicated ones, such as balance poses and poses on the floor that require more advanced flexibility and/or strength. If you practice standing poses regularly you'll notice an almost immediate improvement in your leg and hip flexibility, as well as increased strength and general stability throughout your entire body. Your balance and posture will improve, too.

Warrior Spirit

One of our favorite groups of poses is the group of warrior poses. Because these poses are fun and empowering, they are popular. But don't let the name mislead you!

We tend to think of warriors as wearing armor. In yoga, the warrior represents the strength of openness and the expansion of consciousness. The rosebud makes an appropriate analogy. A rosebud that is not nourished or is pinched off from its source will wither and die. A fully nourished and strong rosebud will open and bloom. Both are fragile flowers, but one of them never realizes its potential. The other does.

When you practice the warrior poses, visualize your entire center holding itself up. This internal lift, while moving into, holding, and out of the warrior poses, strengthens and tones your muscles from the inside out. Also lift your abdomen while in the pose. You can still breathe fully and fully expand your abdomen while you keep it lifted; the lift supports, rather than impedes, the breath. Think strong foundation, lengthened body, fluid movements, easy balance.

Listen to Your Body

We will remind you throughout this book to listen to your body. Pay attention to how your body is responding to each pose. Focus on how you feel, not on something else like the television or the radio. Listening to your body and responding to its needs is the best way to get the most out of each pose.

That's a short overview. Are you ready to begin? Let's stand up and get to it!

The Least You Need to Know

➤ Getting to know yourself better will make yoga better!

➤ Know thyself.

➤ Know thyself.

➤ Know thyself. (... And then it will truly be nice to know you, too!)

➤ Good posture, correct breathing, beginning at the beginning, and a concentrated focus will optimize your yoga workout—and your life!

Part 4

Energize: Postures to Build Strength and Endurance

On to the workout! Part 4 consists of energizing postures you can try, master, and incorporate into your workout. Standing poses build strength, endurance, and steadiness. Balance poses improve poise and self-possession. Backbends release the flow of energy through your body. Twists and inversions rejuvenate and revitalize you.

Vinyasa is a method of yoga that strings postures together in a sequence with deep breathing to create an active, flowing routine full of movement and energy. Depending on which postures you include in your vinyasa, you'll experience a mild to strenuous cardiovascular workout. We show you a few examples, including the well-known and popular sun salutation, then set you free to create your own vinyasa routines. Have fun!

Chapter 13

What Do You Stand For?

So, are you ready to start moving? Great! You may be eager to jump right in and try the headstand or the full lotus position, but learning the basics first is important. You wouldn't be able to play an advanced piano concerto competently without first mastering the scales. In yoga, those "scales" can be likened to the most basic of poses: the mountain pose, from which many standing poses begin.

Tadasana: Mountain Pose

The mountain pose is an important basic pose to learn well. It is deceptively simple in that it appears as easy as standing, but it actually requires great concentration because the entire body must be equally balanced. *Tada* means "mountain," and *sana* means "straight," so *tadasana* (pronounced *tah-DAH-sah-nah*) means standing straight like a mountain. As you stand in *tadasana,* try to feel the firmness and stability of a mountain.

The mountain pose benefits your body in many ways. It helps to maintain balance and posture, which leads to internal balance, which leads to good health. You must have a clear understanding of this pose and be able to hold it well before you can hold any of the other standing poses well—including the headstand, which is really just an upside-down version of *tadasana!*

When holding *tadasana*, it's important to breathe. Let your lower ribs expand on the inhalation. Imagine your diaphragm lowering to make room in your lower chest. You are a soldier of peace in *tadasana*, so there's no need to put up your armor or feel any tension. Try to notice the difference between tension and simple awareness.

As you complete the pose, distribute your weight evenly between your heels and toes, between each leg, over each hip. Think *balance*. Let your belly expand and release its tension with each inhalation.

Ouch!

When holding the mountain pose, be careful to stay balanced. If you stand off-balance, your spine's elasticity and alignment will be compromised. Also, tilt your hips slightly in, which will naturally tilt your stomach back toward your spine. The heels on our shoes (even on our gym shoes!) constantly push our hips back and our stomachs out. Realign them with *tadasana*.

1. Put your feet together with your toes pointed forward. Your arms should hang by your sides with the palms facing toward your body.

2. Lift your toes off the ground. Notice how the arches of your feet feel. Slightly lift up. Now, slowly place your toes back on the ground while you maintain the feeling of the lift in your arches. Feel the lift all the way up your entire body.

3. Feel your spine and the back of your neck lengthening. (Remember that string pulling up the crown of your head?) Pull up the thigh muscles and lift the front of your body. Relax your hands and face.

4. **Yoga Adventure:** Visualization is an effective tool for the mountain pose. As you hold this pose, imagine you are a mountain. Feel how steady, strong, solid, balanced you are. Feel

how you are both a unique, powerful manifestation, and at the same time no different from the planet you rise out of.

5. *Ta Da (sana)!*

Trikonasana: Triangle, the Happy Pose

Forming triangles with your body will teach it a sense of direction. The basic triangle, or *trikonasana* (pronounced *trih-koh-NAH-sah-nah*), is known as the happy pose because it opens your Venus *chakra* (the energy center located behind your heart) and allows joy to fill your body and radiate within you and from you. *Trikonasana* tones your spine and waist. It stimulates your bowels and intestines, strengthens your legs and ankles, improves your circulation, and develops your chest. It also strengthens the breath.

As you come back into *tadasana,* feel your chest opening. Breathe freely and deeply.

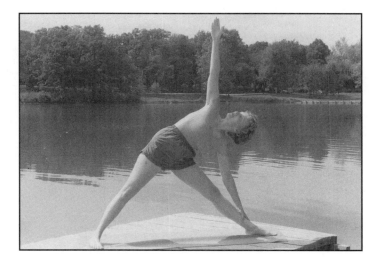

1. Stand with your feet about three feet apart, right foot pointed forward, left foot turned out comfortably, about 90 degrees.
2. Bend to the left, reaching your left arm toward your left foot, and stretching your right arm straight up over your head. If you can, rest your left hand on your left ankle or calf.
3. Look straight ahead or toward the sky and stretch your neck. Feel the triangle formed by your legs and the ground, as well as the rough triangle shape formed by your entire body. Breathe deeply.
4. Slowly come back to a standing position, then repeat on the other side.

5. **Yoga Adventure:** Take the triangle pose a step further with the revolved triangle pose. After holding the pose for a few breaths, switch your arms. Bring the raised arm down, and hold the other side of your calf or ankle. Bring the arm that was holding your calf or ankle straight up above you. Breathe, then return to the mountain pose, and repeat on the other side.

The revolved triangle pose may, upon first glance, look like the regular triangle pose, but look closer. The body is twisted around so the left hand is by the right foot. This is considered a more difficult pose that incorporates a full spinal twist into the triangle.

Wise Yogi Tells Us

In *trikonasana*, don't worry if you can't reach your ankle at first. The length of your stretch doesn't equal the quality of your yoga. Don't be so eager to touch your ankle that you tilt your body forward, cutting off your body's energy flow. Pretend your shoulders must stay pressed against an invisible wall behind you. You'll stay straight and your energy will soar!

Parshvakonasana: Side Angle Stretch

Parshva means "flank" or "side," and *kona* means "angle"—hence, *parshvakonasana* (pronounced *par-shvah-KOH-nah-sah-nah*) means side angle stretch! This pose tones your legs, strengthens your knees, and lengthens your spine. It relieves back pain and sciatica problems, and stretches and strengthens the hips and stomach.

Exhale as you go into this pose, and inhale as you come out; breathe while you hold the pose.

1. Stand with your feet three to four feet apart. Point your left foot forward and turn your right foot out.

2. Bend your right knee into a right angle with the floor and lean into the stretch so that the right side of your body moves toward the top of your right thigh and your right hand reaches toward the ground beside your right foot. Don't worry about touching the floor with your hand. Concentrate on the side stretch of your body.

3. Stretch your left arm over your head so that it forms a relatively straight line with your left leg and torso. Your left palm should face downward. Look up toward your arm and feel the stretch from your toes into your fingertips. Breathe deeply.

4. Return to the mountain pose, then repeat on the other side.

5. **Getting Started:** The side angle stretch feels amazing first thing in the morning when your muscles really need a good stretch to wake up fully. This pose is so energizing that it might eventually replace that cup of coffee!

Ouch!

In the side angle stretch, be careful not to overextend your bent knee. It should be at or nearly at a right angle to the floor. Also, don't let your back leg flop. Keep it active by pushing down on your back heel. If you don't like the smell of your armpit as you look up against your arm, well ... change deodorants! (Hey, at least you're working up a sweat!)

145

Virabhadrasana: Warrior Pose

It takes the tremendous strength of a warrior to "conquer" inner peace. The warrior pose, or *virabhadrasana* (pronounced *vee-rab-hah-DRAH-sah-nah*), fills the body with nobility and strength, calling upon the power and nourishment of the sun while firmly planting the feet upon the earth. *Vira* means "hero" and *bhadra* means "auspicious," so *virabhadrasana* means "heroic auspicious posture." Wow! Didn't you always want to be part *yogi* and part Conan?

We demonstrate three different versions of *virabhadrasana* here: warrior 1, warrior 2, and warrior 3.

Warrior 1

The first warrior pose aids in deep breathing, relieves a stiff neck and shoulders, strengthens the legs, and trims the hips.

Be sure to exhale as you go into the warrior pose, and inhale as you go out of the pose. Think "strength" instead of "tense." Be careful to relax your muscles while in the warrior pose. Keep your face and neck relaxed. Breathe normally. Feel the warrior strength gathering inside you. Strength doesn't come from muscle contraction. Strength comes from the mind.

1. Stand with your feet three to four feet apart. Turn your right foot out, and turn your left foot so that it is facing slightly toward the right foot.

2. Bend your left leg into or close to a right angle and rotate your body to the right, directly in line with the left leg.

3. Raise both arms over your head with your palms facing each other. Look straight ahead or upward at your hands. If your shoulders are relaxed, bring your palms together. For those of us with tight shoulders, it's best to keep the hands apart, which will help the shoulders stay down away from the ears.

4. Keep your back foot firmly planted and your back leg straight. Push down on your back heel. Take three rich, full breaths.

5. Remember that lift of your arches in mountain pose? Notice what happens when you apply that technique here. Lift the toes of the back foot. Watch the arch slightly lift. Slowly place your toes back on the ground while maintaining the lift in the arch. As the toes touch the ground, let the lift of the arch ascend throughout the rest of your body. Breathe.

6. Return to the starting position and repeat on the other side.

7. **Yoga Adventure:** Bring your palms together and interlace your fingers over your head, while keeping your index fingers pointed straight up. Keep your shoulders down, away from your ears. Look up at your hands while keeping your neck strong. Imagine strength and energy shooting out of the tips of your index fingers. This variation intensifies the strength and energy of the warrior 1 pose.

Warrior 2

The second warrior pose has the same benefits as the first, but it also strengthens and shapes the legs, relieves leg cramps, brings flexibility to the legs and back, tones the abdomen, and strengthens the ankles and arms.

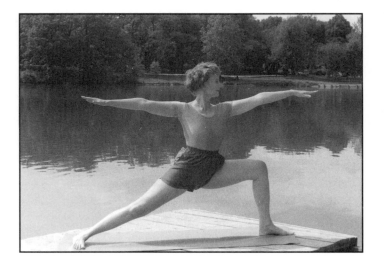

1. Begin as for the warrior 1 pose, but keep your upper body facing forward as you bend your left leg into or close to a right angle with the floor.

2. Lift both arms straight out to form a "T" shape with your body. Look toward your left arm. Keep your shoulders down.

3. Hold the pose for at least a few breaths, return to the starting position, then repeat on the other side.

4. **Yoga Adventure:** Combining warrior 1 and warrior 2 into *vinyasa,* or a flowing sequence, is a great way to get your heart pumping and to energize your body and mind for a challenging day. Begin in the mountain pose, then flow into warrior 1 according to the earlier instructions, then rotate your torso and bring your arms down into the warrior 2 position, then flow back into the mountain. Repeat as many times as you like. Once you've combined these two, add warrior 3 and the lightning bolt pose to the sequence, flowing from warrior 1 to warrior 2 to warrior 3 to lightning bolt back to *tadasana,* then starting all over again. What a way to wake yourself up in the morning! Keep the movements flowing and full of energy. This warrior *vinyasa* is a real confidence builder.

Warrior 3

The warrior 3 position develops the strength and shape of your legs and abdomen; it also gives you agility, poise, better concentration, and improved balance. It is a more difficult pose than the first two warrior poses. Be sure to exhale going into all the warrior poses, and inhale coming out.

1. Assume the warrior 1 pose, then lean forward slightly, slowly straightening your front leg as you lift your back leg.

2. Extend your arms in front of you with your palms together, and look toward your hands. Work toward bringing your arms and lifted leg perpendicular to the floor, but if you can't do that at first, no problem. This is something you will be able to do when you have gained sufficient strength and balance.

3. Return to a neutral position, then repeat on the opposite side.

4. **Yoga Adventure:** How long can you hold this pose? This balance pose is challenging both because you have to balance on one leg and because it takes strength to keep your arms and other leg lifted. Work on extending the amount of time you can hold this pose, for a super-powered, strength-building, balance-honing workout. Watch your breath! As the breath comes into balance, so do the balance poses. Don't hold your breath. Keep breathing, slowly and steadily.

Utkatasana: Lightning Bolt Pose

The lightning bolt pose, or *utkatasana* (pronounced *oot-kah-TAH-sah-nah*), is a powerful pose. *Utkatasana* means "raised posture." As you form the shape of a lightning bolt, you are filled with the dynamic energy of lightning. *Utkatasana* removes shoulder stiffness, strengthens your legs and ankles, lifts your diaphragm, massages your heart, tones your back and stomach, and develops your chest. It also warms up the body.

1. Begin in *tadasana,* the mountain pose.

2. Bend your knees and lift your arms over your head with your palms together or slightly apart. Be careful to keep your knees from buckling inward; keep your feet together, or slightly apart.

3. Extend your arms so they are in line with your torso. Feel the shape of the lightning and breathe deeply. ZAP!

4. Return to *tadasana.*

149

5. **Yoga Adventure:** Vary the lightning bolt pose by turning it into a "squat on heels and toes" pose. Stand with your feet hip-distance apart. Squat, first standing on your toes, then rocking back on your heels. This variation develops the ankles, knees, and arches. Be careful to keep your knees over your ankles. Don't let them droop in or out as you bend. This further strengthens the quadriceps and ankles.

Moving into the "squat on heels and toes" pose.

Balance Poses

We've emphasized before that balance is extremely important in the practice of yoga. When your body is balanced, a connection is formed between the two sides of your body (*ha* and *tha*, as in *Hatha Yoga*). But balance poses do more than coordinate your left and right sides. They help tie your entire body and mind together into a more integrated and fully functioning whole. Balance poses also increase self-confidence, because they teach you to stay centered, calm, and strong in precarious circumstances. If you accomplished the warrior 3 pose in the earlier section, remember how great you felt? That's just a taste of the power of balance poses.

Vrikshasana: *Tree Pose*

Vrikshasana (pronounced *vrik-SHAH-sah-nah*) is one of the most basic balance poses. *Vriksha* means "tree," and a tree is soundly rooted in the earth but grows upward with branches reaching out to the sun. Wind may move the branches, but the tree stands firm. *Vrikshasana* tones the legs, opens the hips, and promotes physical balance. It also develops concentration and mindfulness.

Throughout *vrikshasana*, keep your breathing steady and regular so it doesn't interfere with your balance.

1. Begin in *tadasana*, the mountain pose.

2. Bring your hands together in front of your chest with your palms together (as if you were praying).

3. Bring your left leg up and balance the sole of your left foot on the inner thigh of your right leg, as high as you are able. If it's been a "vida loca" kind of day and you have a hard time balancing on one foot, keep your toes on the ground, turn your one knee out to open the hips, then simply balance the heel against your ankle. It's amazing how calming and balancing this pose can be!

4. Raise your arms over your head, keeping your palms together.

5. Return to *tadasana*, then repeat with the right leg.

Ouch!

In *vrikshasana*, be careful not to raise one hip higher than the other. Keep your hips even by lowering the position of your foot on your inner thigh. Bend your straight knee slightly. If you become aware that you are hyper-extending it, then, with awareness, stop hyper-extending the knee: Straighten it with awareness. If your knees are sore after doing this pose, you probably are hyper-extending.

151

6. **Getting Started:** If you find it too difficult to balance in *tadasana,* you can vary the pose slightly. Bring the sole of your foot to your opposite leg's inner calf instead of the thigh, or even rest it against your opposite ankle, to get a more secure feeling of the balance before hiking that foot all the way up to the opposite thigh. Also, you can leave your palms apart when you raise your arms. This great separation between your hands can help you balance more easily. When you feel more confident in the pose, you can bring that foot up and those palms together.

Ardha Baddha Padmottanasana: *Standing Half Bound Lotus Pose*

The purpose of this more advanced variation of the tree pose is to keep the trunk steady with the help of your arm. It has the same benefits as the tree pose but allows you to open your hips more fully, which in turn opens the Jupiter *chakra* (the energy center located on your spine behind your pelvis). It also allows a fuller chest expansion.

Don't be frustrated if you have trouble getting into the standing half bound lotus pose. If your hips are not open enough yet and your knee isn't pointing toward the floor, it'll be difficult to connect your hand with your foot and could also overstrain your knee. Give yourself time and keep practicing the regular tree pose. Eventually your body will accommodate you.

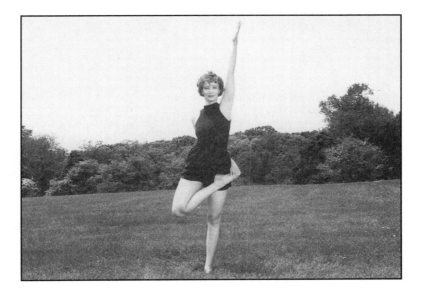

1. The standing half bound lotus is similar to the tree pose, except your bent right ankle rests on the front of your straight left thigh.

2. Bring your right arm behind your back and connect it to your right foot in front.

3. Lower your knee slightly toward the floor and raise your left arm over your head. Take three breaths.

4. Return to the starting position, then repeat on the other side.

5. **Getting Started:** This is a challenging pose and not for beginners. Poses that open the chest and increase shoulder and spinal flexibility will help get you to a point where you can reach your arm far enough behind you to grab your foot. Practice the eagle pose (following), side angle stretch (earlier in this chapter), bow pose and upward facing dog (Chapter 14), and both standing and lying down spinal twists (Chapter 15) to help your body prepare for the half bound lotus.

Garudasana: *Eagle*

The eagle is a god in Indian mythology, and so is considered sacred and important. As with the tree pose, *garudasana* (pronounced *gah-roo-DAH-sah-nah*) improves balance and concentration as well as develops the ankles and removes stiffness in the shoulders. Symbolically, the eagle represents the life force/*prana*.

1. Begin in *tadasana*, but with the knees slightly bent.

2. Bend one leg over the other like you are crossing your thighs, then hook your ankle around the back of your other ankle. Try to stay balanced between your heel and toe.

153

3. Bend your elbows and bring one arm under the other arm, connecting your palms in front of your face. Even though your body is twisting every which way, imagine your torso lifting and straightening. Breathe!

4. Return to *tadasana,* and repeat on the other side. This pose is usually easier going one way than it is going the other way, but try it both ways and eventually you'll balance.

5. **Getting Started:** The eagle pose is a challenging pose. Don't force that ankle around your standing leg, or you could injure your knee! If your ankle doesn't hook around your standing leg easily, just place the top of your foot behind the ankle or calf of your standing leg. Eventually your flexibility will increase. Better to work within your own limits than to injure yourself!

Plank Pose

The plank pose develops strength in your arms and legs. It helps to create a balanced and strong body. It is often used as a transition pose, leading or connecting one pose to another.

1. Lie on your stomach, with your fingertips in line with your shoulders and your elbows bent in toward the body, toes curled under.

2. Push yourself up into an extended pushup position (the "up" end of the pushup) and hold.

3. Try to keep your body in a straight line from ears to ankles. You will discover where the weakest sections of your body are the longer you hold this position: They are the parts that start to sag toward the floor!

4. Breathe. Push your heels out to keep your lower back from caving in.

5. Come back down onto your stomach, or use this pose as a transition into the following arm balance pose.

Vashishthasana: *Arm Balance*

Vashishthasana (pronounced *VAH-shish-THAH-sah-nah*) is a pose named after the Indian sage Vashishtha. *Vashishthasana* strengthens the wrists and arms, and tones the lumbar and coccyx regions of the spine. It also develops concentration, nonattachment to either achievement or failure, and an undisturbed, steady mind.

Ouch!

Keep breathing steadily throughout *vashishthasana*. Don't let your hips droop down, because this will cause strain to your back and put undue force on your arms. Keep your elbows straight and keep your foot balanced on your leg. Don't let anything droop!

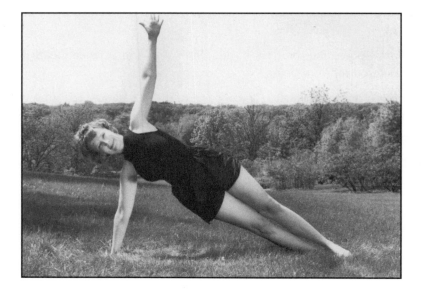

1. Begin in the plank pose.

2. Turn your entire body to the right, and balance on your right arm and foot on the side of your body. Your torso should be in a straight line, held in a diagonal to the floor by your right arm.

155

3. Lift your left arm up straight in the air with your palm facing forward.

4. **Getting Started:** Don't lock your elbow in this pose, or you could injure it. Keep your arm straight, but keep strength and flexibility in your elbow so you could bend it easily at any time during the pose (just as you would keep your knees just slightly bent rather than locked when standing for a long time). Your muscles should be holding your weight, not your elbow joint. And when you feel you can't hold your own weight for another second? For goodness's sake, stop!

Learning the basic standing postures is a great way to start, and balance poses will increase your stability. Practicing these basics will improve all aspects of your yoga practice and give you an inner peace and strength.

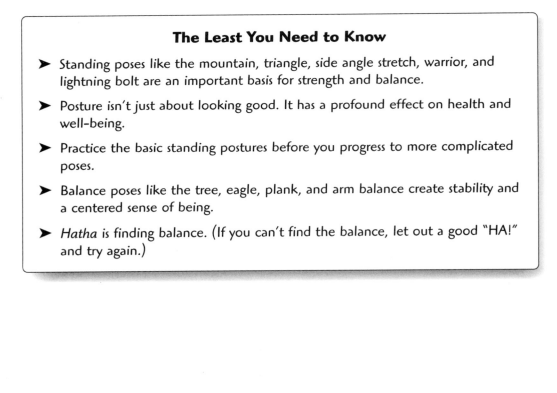

The Least You Need to Know

➤ Standing poses like the mountain, triangle, side angle stretch, warrior, and lightning bolt are an important basis for strength and balance.

➤ Posture isn't just about looking good. It has a profound effect on health and well-being.

➤ Practice the basic standing postures before you progress to more complicated poses.

➤ Balance poses like the tree, eagle, plank, and arm balance create stability and a centered sense of being.

➤ *Hatha* is finding balance. (If you can't find the balance, let out a good "HA!" and try again.)

Chapter 14

Bending Over Backbends

In This Chapter

➤ The health benefits of backbends

➤ Backbends help you laugh more

➤ Lots of great backbending postures to try: cobra, bow, upward facing dog, fish, camel, and wheel

➤ Modifications, challenges, and other tips to improve your yoga practice

A few people have naturally flexible spines and find backbends easy, but for most people, backbends are a challenge. We tend to spend more of our lives bent slightly forward, and our spines just aren't used to bending the other way. All the more reason to practice backbends—for the sake of balance.

Open Up and Laugh More

Whether or not you are naturally flexible, bending poses are extremely beneficial for improving your spine and toning your internal organs. The movement into and the holding of backbends releases your *chakras,* or the energy centers in your body, so energy and joy can flow through you unimpeded. (See Chapter 20, "*Chakras, Mudras, Mantras,* and *Mandalas.*") After a few good backbends, you may just laugh out loud.

Start by performing a simple stretch to open your neck, shoulders, and chest. Just like the figure in the following drawing, sit up straight in a chair and begin to arch your neck back. Inhale as you do it. Focus your gaze upward. Feel that openness in the center of your chest? It's as if you're lifting your heart—and your spirits as well! It's important to arch your neck only as far as you can support it, as in the first window in the drawing. Try forcing your lower lip over your upper lip, as you see in the second window. It's hard to frown in a backbending posture! Again, in backbends, you always want to be supported; avoid the impulse to crunch your neck back as the figure is doing in the third window of the drawing. A crunched neck (a crunched *anything,* for that matter) is very anti-yoga and can lead to discomfort and injury. Now *smile.* Doesn't it feel good?

Let's get bent!

Opening stretch before bending. Avoid crunching your neck as the figure in the third box is doing!

Bhujangasana: Cobra Pose

Bhujanga means "serpent," and the cobra is a sacred and revered serpent in India. But what is a serpent? Basically, one big spine! In the cobra pose, *bhujangasana* (pronounced *BOO-jhan-GAH-sah-nah*), concentrate on allowing the strength of your spine to move you. The cobra pose helps to align your spinal disks, open up your heart *chakra,* and strengthen your back. It also strengthens your nervous system and your eyes.

When practicing the cobra pose, keep your elbows in toward the body. As your shoulders rise off the floor, don't scrunch them up around your neck. Keep your eyes open and peering up to tone your peripheral vision (typically the first part of the eyesight to degenerate).

The cobra pose.

1. Lie on your stomach, flat on the floor, with your heels and toes together. Place your hands on the floor on either side of your chest. Rest your forehead on the floor (you might want to use a mat for this one).

2. Inhale and lift your forehead, then chin, then shoulders, then chest off the floor. Keep your hips pressed against the floor.

3. Look upward and breathe. Try sticking out your tongue and opening your mouth wide to help release your face. Then return to the starting position.

4. **Yoga Adventure:** Does a snake have arms? Of course not! You shouldn't rely on your arms for this pose. To see how much you are using your arms as a support, lift your palms off the floor, as you see in the second figure in the drawing. How much of your body comes down? If it's a lot, your arms are doing a good portion of the work. Don't go up so high just yet. Let your spine do the work.

A Yoga Minute

Some doctors believe many cases of back pain are psychologically caused. Deep stress or emotional problems may manifest themselves as a backache.

Dhanurasana: Bow Pose

Dhanurasana (pronounced *DAH-noo-RAH-sah-nah*), a.k.a., the bow pose, is a high-energy pose. Imagine your body is like an archer's bow ready to launch an arrow. This pose keeps your spine supple, tones your abdomen, massages your back muscles, strengthens your concentration, and decreases laziness.

When in the bow pose, be sure to grab your ankles, not your toes or feet. If you can't grab your ankles, simply bring your hands back as far as you can alongside your body. Move your hands toward your ankles, *not* your ankles toward your hands. Keep your elbows straight, not bent, and don't lift your shoulders up to your ears—keep them pressed down.

The bow pose.

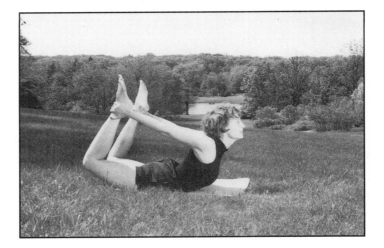

1. Lie on your stomach. Bring both arms behind you and bend both knees.
2. Grasp your ankles with your hands.
3. Pull your body so it lengthens like a bow, and look up. Hold for two or three breaths.

Half Bow

In the half bow, the bow is strung one string at a time. When in the half bow, be careful not to lean over to the side that is held straight. Balance both sides of your body. Be sure to breathe. You'll be able to tell how much caffeine you've had lately by how much your straight hand shakes!

The half bow pose.

1. Begin on your stomach as with the bow pose, but extend your left arm straight over your head, palm down.

2. Bend your right knee and bring your right arm back toward your right ankle.

3. Push your stomach into the floor with your tailbone tipped toward the floor. Lift your head and chest. Keep your focus on the outstretched arm.

4. **Getting Started:** This pose may look easier than the full bow pose, but don't be fooled. You need the same concentration as with the bow pose. This pose is a preparation for the bow pose, so hold it for only a few breaths on each side. Then try going into full bow pose for a longer sail!

Rocking Bow

The rocking bow is the full bow plus! It aids digestion, relieves constipation, and tones the intestines. The fuller the bow, the easier it is to rock and roll!

The rocking bow pose.

1. Get into the bow pose.

2. Using your breath, rock your body back and forth. Inhale as the body rocks back, exhale forward. Keep your arms straight.

3. **Yoga Adventure:** This high-energy, aerobic pose-in-motion is great for your whole body. Pick your favorite song with a medium-to-slow beat and see if you can rock and roll through the whole thing. If not, you can work up to it as you get fitter.

Wise Yogi Tells Us

Swami Vishnu Devananda says, "OM is a bow, the arrow is the Soul, Brahman is the arrow's goal." Backbends are so good at making it easier to breathe deeply—by opening up the chest and abdomen—that many people crave backbends! The deep breathing gets more oxygen to the brain. As a result, you feel stimulated, refreshed, and energized. Get a double benefit by completing your yoga backbends with a few balancing forward bends to relax the spine, along with a few moments of meditation on the *swami*'s words.

Urdhvamukha Shvanasana: Upward Facing Dog

Urdhva means "upward," and *mukha* means "mouth" or "face." *Shvan* means "dog." *Urdhvamukha Shvanasana* (pronounced OORD-vah-MOOK-hah shvah-NAH-sahn-ah) looks like a dog stretching upward. (Yoga shows great respect for dog poses—after all, what is "dog" spelled backward?) Upward facing dog is great for a stiff back. It strengthens the spine, alleviates backaches, increases respiration and circulation (especially to the pelvic area), and strengthens the eyes.

The upward facing dog pose.

162

1. Go into the cobra pose, then inhale further and straighten your arms, keeping your back legs strong (this takes the pressure off your back).

2. Inhale and lift the front of your body off the floor as you look up. Continue to lift so your hips and legs are held just slightly off the floor, too. Your hands and the tops of your feet are the only parts of your body making contact with the floor in this advanced version. Let your arms do much of the work, not just your spine (as in the cobra pose).

3. Exhale as you come back down to the floor.

Matsyasana: Go Fish

A fish must open its gills to breathe; *matsyasana* (pronounced *mahtz-YAH-sah-nah*) fills the lungs with air, improving the *yogi*'s ability to float in water (try it!). The fish pose energizes the calcium-regulating parathyroid gland (located in your neck), strengthens the abdomen, improves the voice by opening the Mercury *chakra* located in the throat (see Chapter 20), and relieves mental tension.

Ouch!

Be careful not to let your legs roll in while in upward facing dog. Lift your inner legs. If you feel off-balance, concentrate on centering your balance on your feet. Weak legs will cause your back to curve in and hurt. Keep them strong! Don't bend your elbows or knees.

Half Fish Pose

The half fish pose is a simpler version of the full fish pose that follows. Start with this pose and work your way up to the full fish!

In the half fish pose, don't let your feet fall to the side. Keep your knees straight. Make sure the top of your head, not the back of your head, rests on the floor. Keep your elbows in, breathe regularly, and don't put your weight on your head. Let your elbows and arms support your weight.

1. Lie flat on your back with your feet together and your knees straight.

2. Place your palms facing down under your tailbone with your thumbs touching.

3. Inhale, then lift your upper chest and arch your back, supporting your weight with your arms and elbows. Allow your head to tilt back.

4. Rest the top of your head lightly on the floor. Feel the strength of the lift in your arms and chest. Hold for three breaths, then exhale as you come down.

5. **Getting Started:** If you have a stiff neck, jaw, or upper back, or if you feel uncomfortable resting your head in this position for any reason, place a folded towel, blanket, or bolster-type pillow under your neck and gently look up and

163

back, to accustom your neck and head to this position. No need to rush into the full tilt before you feel ready!

The half fish pose.

Full Fish Pose

This pose is the same as the half fish pose, except your legs and feet are in the full lotus position (see Chapter 17, "Are You Sitting Down?") and your hands hold your feet. If you cannot do the full lotus, simply cross your legs. Your hands do not need to hold your feet if you aren't in full lotus position. This variation further opens the pelvis and promotes energy flow through all your *chakras*.

1. Lie down on your back and bring your knees up, then cross your legs into the lotus pose, with each foot lying sole-up on top of the opposite thigh (see Chapter 17). Or, if you haven't worked up to this pose yet, simply cross your legs.

The full fish pose.

2. As you bring your crossed legs down to the ground, arch your back up. Let your head relax backward; the top of your head just brushes the ground or floor.

3. Reach your hands toward your feet, and if you can, hold your feet. If you can't reach your feet, place your palms on your thighs. The body is fully balanced in this position and does not need the additional arm strength as in half-fish pose.

4. Breathe deeply in this position as your lungs are fully expanded.

5. Bring your knees and head up, uncross your legs, and straighten them out. Lift your head up and release the arch in your back. Lie with a flat back. Rest on your back for a few minutes.

6. **Getting Started:** This pose is difficult because your arms don't support your body weight. If you don't feel comfortable about resting the top of your head against the floor without your arms for support (in other words, if you don't feel your back and neck are strong enough to support you), use your arms as you did in the half fish, while still keeping your legs crossed.

Wise Yogi Tells Us

Whenever a particular pose opens a *chakra*, concentrate on that area while holding the pose. Feel the energy flowing through and from the target *chakra*. Your mind can help open your *chakras* even further. See Chapter 20 for an introduction to *chakras*.

Ustrasana: Camel

Ustra means "camel," and *ustrasana* (pronounced *oohs-TRAH-sah-nah*) imitates the hump of a camel. Your shoulders and chest become more open and mobile through the camel pose. Your abdomen is stretched, digestion is improved, rib muscles are strengthened, and the pose can also help *sciatica* (a painful condition felt in the hip or thigh, resulting from inflammation of the *sciatic nerve*—a long nerve that starts in the hip and runs down the back of the leg).

When practicing the camel pose, pretend there is a wall in front of you and you are pressing your thighs toward it. Bend only as far backward as you can while keeping your neck properly supported by your neck muscles.

1. Begin on your knees with your feet behind you, legs and feet together or slightly apart.

2. Stretch your hips and thighs forward as you reach behind you with your arms. Pretend there is a wall in front of you and your thighs stay pressed against the wall. The spine extends and lifts up as you lean back.

3. Let your body bend backward and your head tilt back. Look up. If you can't reach your heels, eventually you will. Take it gradually.

The camel pose.

4. Take several deep breaths in the pose, then exhale as you release and come forward to the beginning position.

5. **Getting Started:** If this pose is too difficult, you can place a chair or a footstool behind you and use it to support your elbows or hands (depending on the height of your support) behind you. Remember not to let your head hang loosely, but to support it with your neck muscles as you look up.

Cakrasana: Doin' Wheelies!

Cakrasana (pronounced *chah-KRAH-sah-nah*) makes your body strong and mobile, like a wheel. It stretches and strengthens the stomach, improves the concentration by bringing blood to the head, and gives greater control over the body. It also prevents bad posture, tones the extremities, improves the memory, heightens energy and vitality, brings a feeling of lightness to the body, and improves circulation to the trachea and larynx. (The *trachea*—also known as the windpipe—is the passageway between the larynx and the lungs, and the *larynx* is the area of the throat that contains the vocal cords.)

In the wheel pose, your hips may feel too tight to lengthen sufficiently. If your shoulders are tight or your arms are weak, you may be unable to push yourself up into position. Just keep working at it, and one day … POW! There it is.

The wheel pose.

1. Lie flat on your back with your knees bent, feet flat on the floor.
2. Bend your elbows toward the sky and bring your palms to the floor next to your ears, fingers facing your feet.
3. Lift your navel (think of lifting your Mars *chakra,* located behind your navel), and push your torso up into an arch using your arms and legs. Your body will form an arch shape, and your head should be off the floor, your arms and legs almost straight.
4. Hold for as long as is comfortable, then gently come back down.
5. **Getting Started:** If the full wheel pose is too difficult, you can modify the position. In this variation, the stomach remains flat and the elbows and knees stay bent, so you aren't pushing yourself all the way up. You can leave your head resting on the floor between your hands.

Know Your Sanskrit

The wheel pose is the most dynamic of backbends. It's the one that effectively stimulates all of the *chakras* (or *cakras*). Hence the name of the pose: ***cakrasana.***

Backbends can help you laugh more ... and better! Don't we all need more and better laughs?

The Least You Need to Know

➤ Backbending poses are important for increasing flexibility, as well as keeping various internal organs open and free.

➤ Open, toned organs result in open *chakras* and a free flow of energy throughout the body.

➤ Backbends are great for people who work at desks or computers all day; they correct that hunched-over posture.

➤ Backbends make it easier to breathe deeply and fully; they stimulate the body and get more oxygen to the brain.

Chapter 15

Come on, Body, Let's Do the Twist

In This Chapter

➤ Gentle twists to realign your spine

➤ Inversions to invigorate

➤ Spinal twists to scintillate

➤ Modifications, challenges, and other tips to improve your yoga practice

Twists are wonderful ways to clear out your system. They free and realign your spine so that every part of your body works better. Twists massage the internal organs and help the body force toxins out to be carried away for elimination. *Prana* is allowed to enter the spine and energize it. For balance, always remember to do *both* sides of a spinal twist.

And talk about a fountain of youth—inversions are amazing postures that balance all that standing and walking around right-side-up. Blood flows to the brain, gravity works the other way on every part of your body—in fact, after a good headstand, you'll feel almost like you've spent the day at a spa. So get ready to break out of the old habit of existing upright!

Maricyasana: Spinal Twist

Maricyasana (pronounced *MAH-rih-si-AH-sah-nah*) gives the spine a nice, lateral stretch, increasing spinal elasticity. The spinal twist also improves side-to-side mobility; decreases backaches and hip pain; contracts and tones the liver, spleen, and intestines; reduces abdominal size; improves the nervous system; prevents calcification at the base of the spine; frees the joints; and rouses your *kundalini* energy (see Chapter 5, "Going Back in Time: The Yoga Tradition"). Whew! It's energizing just saying all that!

The spinal twist.

1. Sit on the floor with both legs out in front of you.

2. Bend your left leg over the outside of your right leg, then turn to the left.

Ouch!

In the spinal twist, don't over-twist your neck. Keep the twist the full length of the spine for full benefit. Some people over-twist the neck and neglect the full twist of the spine. Keep your bent knee facing up to support a steady twist of the spine.

3. Bend your right arm and place your right elbow on the outside of your left knee. Keep your shoulders down.

4. Lift your spine and twist, looking behind you as you push your chest forward (in the direction you are facing) to lengthen the spine.

5. Return to the starting position and repeat on the other side.

6. **Getting Started:** The movement of the spinal twist should be slow and deliberate, no matter how advanced you are. If you whip your spine around to the side, you could throw your vertebrae out of alignment. If you are having trouble getting the feel of it, count out five seconds as you twist around to look behind you, then take five seconds to twist back to center, five seconds to twist in the other direction, and so on.

Bound Knee Spinal Twist

This variation opens your hips as the spinal twist does, but be sure to keep your back straight and shoulders down. And remember to enjoy this pose. If you aren't enjoying this pose, skip it for now and try a different spinal twist instead. This is a more advanced twist.

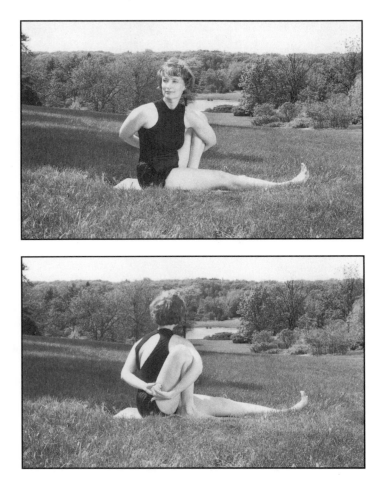

The bound knee spinal twist.

1. From a sitting position with your legs straight out in front of you, bend your left knee and bring your heel in, right up against your body.

2. Turn to your right, bringing the left shoulder around the left knee.

3. Bring your right arm behind your back and connect your hands.

4. **Getting Started:** Can't quite connect your hands? Just reach them toward each other. You'll get there eventually. No hurry! As your shoulders open, your reach will expand, too.

Lying Down Spinal Twist

This variation tones the spine and strengthens the legs. It can also be quite relaxing as gravity helps you out.

The lying down spinal twist.

1. Begin by lying down, with your knees bent and your palms together in front of your chest, as if in prayer (*namaste*).

2. Straighten your arms toward the sky, and let your knees and outstretched arms drop (control the movement) to the right.

3. Lift your left arm, and bring it up and over, so it rests on your left side. Your arms are extended like a "t" with your body. Gently turn your head and look at your left hand.

4. Breathe. Enjoy. Relax.

5. Turn your head back to the right, bring your left hand back to your right hand, then gently bring your knees back to center.

6. Repeat on the other side.

7. **Yoga Adventure:** For an extra challenge, practice deep breathing while resting in the lying down spinal twist. The twist adds resistance to the expansion of the lungs, strengthening all the muscles used for breathing.

Setu Bandha Sarvangasana: **Bridge Pose**

Yes, *setu bandha sarvangasana* (pronounced *SAY-too BAHN-dah SAHR-vahn-GAH-sah-nah*) looks like a bridge. *Setu* means "bridge," and *sarvangasana* is composed of *sarva* (all), *anga* (limb), and of course, *asana* (posture). *Setu bandha sarvangasana* also strengthens the neck and back; tones the entire spine; builds supple wrists; and bathes the pituitary, thyroid, and adrenal glands in blood and other nutrients. The bridge pose helps intestinal function as well. This pose is a good preliminary to the shoulderstand.

The bridge pose.

1. Lie flat on the floor, with your knees bent and your feet flat on the floor, about hip-distance apart. Keep your hands to your sides.

2. Grab hold of your ankles and bring them directly under your bent knees. Lift your hips, creating a bridge shape. Place your hands under your lower back for support, pointing your fingers in toward your spine. Keep your elbows next to your body. Your head, neck, and shoulders should stay on the floor.

3. Tighten the buttocks muscles to support your lifted torso. Make sure your knees are aligned with your ankles, that they face forward, and that they don't fall in or out as you hold the pose.

The half bridge pose.

4. **Getting Started:** If the bridge pose is too difficult, start with a half bridge pose. Clasp your hands under your body, drawing your elbows in so your arms are

straight and resting on the floor underneath you. Concentrate on lifting your body as high as you can. This pose builds strength and flexibility to prepare your body for the full bridge pose.

The extended bridge pose.

5. **Yoga Adventure:** For an even greater strength challenge, try the extended bridge pose. Walk your feet out, away from your body, until your legs are straight. Keep those abdominals lifted and buttocks muscles working—you don't want your bridge to sag! The extended bridge is a very difficult pose that takes a lot of torso strength. Be kind to your back. If it hurts, you shouldn't do it. Remember yoga's first principle? *Ahimsa*—nonviolence. We are shaping our bodies into postures nonviolently. Through this process, we build bridges of peace!

Sarvangasana: Shoulderstand

Sarvangasana (pronounced *SAHR-vahn-GAH-sah-nah*) is a great inversion that stimulates the thyroid gland and the Mercury *chakra* (located in the throat). It reverses the pull of gravity on your internal organs and reduces the strain on your heart, because your heart doesn't have to work as hard to pump to the extremities when inverted. The shoulderstand helps with varicose veins; purifies the blood; nourishes the brain, lungs, and heart; strengthens the eyesight; and is a great headache remedy.

The shoulderstand.

1. Lie flat on the floor, then bring both legs and hips up in the air. Lift up by contracting your abdominal and buttocks muscles; don't just swing your legs up. Although a little bit of a swing can help you get up there, let your muscles do most of the work.

2. Support your lower back with your hands so your upper arms are resting on the floor behind you, your elbows are bent, and your hands rest on your back with your fingers facing inward, toward your spine.

3. Bring your shoulders away from your ears, and push your feet toward the ceiling, almost as if you were hanging by your feet. Breathe! (You'll probably notice that breathing feels different upside down.)

4. **Getting Started:** If you can't get up into a shoulderstand, don't force it. First practice the shoulderstand by bringing your legs back, as in the first drawing, then holding there for a while to accustom your body to the inversion. To protect your neck, it is best to go up into a full shoulderstand, especially the first time, under the guidance of an instructor. Typical problems during a shoulderstand are the tendency to crunch the neck, hold the breath, and twist the neck. Think of your neck lengthening as you hold the pose. Put a folded towel or blanket under your neck, right at the tip of your shoulders. Breathe! Don't allow your elbows to slide outward, and keep your neck lengthened and your feet together.

Halasana: **Plough Pose**

Halasana (pronounced *hah-LAH-sah-nah*) looks like a plough, and *hala* means "plough." The plough pose stimulates the spine; strengthens the nervous system; improves the circulation; releases neck tension; relieves constipation; decreases insomnia; promotes mental relaxation; activates the Mercury *chakra* (in the throat); improves communication; and stimulates the stomach, spleen, small intestine, heart, liver, gall bladder, and kidneys.

The plough pose.

1. Lie on your back with your knees bent, feet flat on the floor, and hands at your waist.

175

2. Inhale and raise your legs, hips, and buttocks off the ground, as you did for the shoulderstand. But this time, instead of bringing your feet up, curl backward, keeping your legs straight.

3. Exhale, and lower your feet to the floor behind your head. Touch your legs to the ground only when they are straight and you feel no strain in your neck.

4. Clasp your hands under your body, facing away from your feet.

5. **Getting Started:** In the plough pose, be sure to keep your knees straight. Don't twist your head or neck. It helps to learn from a teacher or experienced *yogi* before you try it. Don't force your toes to the ground; let gravity do this slowly. If your toes seem like they aren't even close, try the plough pose with a cushion or pillow behind you, so your feet can rest on something a little higher.

6. **Yoga Adventure:** For an even greater challenge in the plough pose, try the hands-to-feet variation. This variation is identical to the first plough, except that you stretch your arms along the ground until they touch your feet. This pose further opens and stretches the shoulders. Notice that this looks like an upside-down forward bend? In fact, you can begin to notice that many "different" poses are really the same, just gravitationally different. (Meditate on that for a while!)

The hands to feet pose is a variation of the plough pose.

Shirshasana: Headstand

Shirshasana (pronounced *sher-SHAH-sahn-ah*) is probably one of the most famous yoga poses and is considered the king or queen of the *Hatha Yoga* poses. It stimulates the whole system, improving circulation and strengthening the nervous system, emotions, and brain. Plus, when your body is ready for it, it's fun!

But be sure your body is ready. You must have sufficient arm, shoulder, neck, and stomach strength, plus be well-versed at *tadasana* (remember back in Chapter 13, "What Do You Stand For?"), the mountain pose, so you can balance your weight evenly while upside down. Otherwise, your neck will hurt. Too much pressure on your head is not good! Your weight should be supported by your arms, shoulders, and the strength of your abdomen. The strength of these areas is developed in standing poses. Develop yourself on your feet before standing on your head.

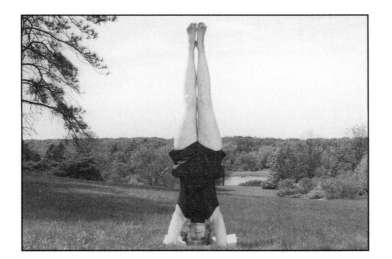

The headstand.

1. Get down on your hands and knees. Grab your left elbow with your right hand and your right elbow with your left hand.

2. Bring your elbows to the ground and release the hold of your hands. Keep your elbows this distance apart for best support.

3. Interlace your fingers so your arms form a point, then cup the top of your head in your palms at the top of the point, as if your head were inside the apex of a triangle.

4. Slowly walk your feet in toward your body, straightening your back, then slowly raise your feet into the air.

5. Breathe! Try to stay balanced in the headstand for at least a few even breaths. Then come back down slowly. Remain with your head down for a few minutes before sitting up.

Ouch!

As wonderful a pose as the headstand is, it shouldn't be practiced under certain circumstances. If you have high blood pressure, heart problems, or are pregnant, don't attempt the headstand or any of the inverted poses. You may still be able to do inversions with no problem, but talk to your yoga-friendly doctor first.

6. **Getting Started:** Balancing in a headstand isn't just a matter of lifting your feet up and hanging out for a while—as your proficiency increases, so does your awareness. Your entire body will be making minor adjustments, tiny movements, little shifts here and there—along your arms, shoulders, hands, neck, back, and legs—to keep you balanced. Notice how your body tries to compensate to keep you balanced. Your body knows. Learn from it!

7. **Yoga Adventure:** For a really advanced pose, try *padma shirshasana* (pronounced *PAHD-mah sher-SHAH-sah-nah*), the lotus headstand; while in the headstand, bring your feet into the full lotus position. (Don't worry, we'll get to that in Chapter 17, "Are You Sitting Down?") To do this pose, which really opens the hips, you must first be very comfortable in the lotus pose and in the headstand. This is definitely an advanced posture. Find a qualified teacher for personal guidance on this one, okay?

Wise Yogi Tells Us

When first attempting the headstand, use a wall for support. The more comfortable and strong you become, the less you'll need the wall, until soon you'll be doing headstands anytime, anywhere!

The lotus headstand—a challenging headstand variation.

Adho Mukha Vrksasana: Handstand

In *adho mukha vrksasana* (pronounced *AHD-hoh MOOK-hah vrik-SHAH-sah-nah*), *adho mukha* means "face down," and *vrksa* means "tree," so just as headstand is mountain pose upside down, handstand is tree pose upside down. To properly perform this "face-down tree" pose or handstand, your arms must be strong. Practice the downward facing dog pose (*adho mukha svanasana*, described in Chapter 18, "Take the Forward Path") to develop your arms and prepare your body for the handstand.

The handstand gives you tremendous energy. It strengthens your arms and shoulders, plus gives you all the blood-cleansing effects of inversions. If trying this pose scares you, work with a partner who can spot you. The handstand, however, requires a lot of combined abdominal and upper-body strength. If you're not strong enough, concentrate on perfecting headstand poses and the downward facing dog pose.

Inversions can be incredibly refreshing and invigorating. Twists also keep the spine flexible and youthful, so dive into this yoga fountain of youth … head first!

Moving from the downward facing dog pose into a handstand.

1. Perform downward facing dog (see Chapter 18) in front of a wall, as the *yogi* is doing in the drawing. Place your hands on the floor, shoulder-width apart, and about three to five inches from the wall. Slowly walk your legs in toward the wall.

2. Exhale and lift one leg straight up. Follow quickly with the other. Keep your arms and legs straight and firm. Push your shoulders away from the floor, and rest your outstretched legs lightly against the wall.

179

3. Hold the pose for as long as is comfortable. Breathe! Exhale as you come down.

4. **Yoga Adventure:** If you are a very experienced *yogi* who can balance easily in a handstand, try this pose without a wall. But don't try this unsupported pose prematurely. Falling over the wrong way could cause you serious injury. If you do start to fall, bend your knees and roll out of the fall safely.

Now you have some basic (and some advanced) poses under your belt. Having fun? We are! But we have more fun in store, in the way of flow poses, or *vinyasa*. Read on to learn how to string yoga poses together in a continuous flow.

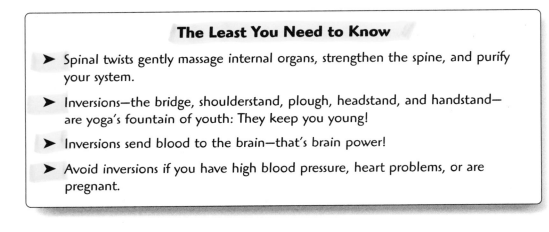

The Least You Need to Know

➤ Spinal twists gently massage internal organs, strengthen the spine, and purify your system.

➤ Inversions—the bridge, shoulderstand, plough, headstand, and handstand— are yoga's fountain of youth: They keep you young!

➤ Inversions send blood to the brain—that's brain power!

➤ Avoid inversions if you have high blood pressure, heart problems, or are pregnant.

Chapter 16

A Continuous Flow

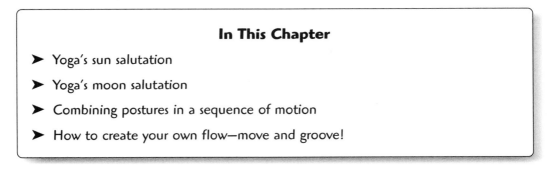

In This Chapter

➤ Yoga's sun salutation

➤ Yoga's moon salutation

➤ Combining postures in a sequence of motion

➤ How to create your own flow—move and groove!

You're probably convinced by now that yoga can be tough and challenging to your strength and flexibility. But what about working up a *real* sweat? That's where *vinyasa* (pronounced *vin-YAH-sah*) comes in! *Vinyasa* combines a series of yoga postures into a long, fluid, unified movement. Poses are held within a *vinyasa,* but the difference is that when you come out of one posture, you flow immediately into another posture. The right flow will give you a great workout, in addition to improving your balance, grace, speed, strength, and agility.

Sweat with the Rhythm

Continuous-flow sequences of yoga postures can be an invigorating cardiovascular workout. Repeating a series of postures in quick succession takes stamina and good lung capacity. A more slowly executed series of poses is also challenging, allowing you to enter each pose fully and deliberately while still engaging in continuous move-ment, making *vinyasa* into a moving meditation.

However you choose to practice yoga postures in a continuous flow, let the rhythm of your body and your breath move you to new levels of mind/body awareness.

Breathe to the Beat

Breath is extremely important in *vinyasa*. Connecting posture to posture and movement to movement is more than just moving muscles. Every movement and every position of a *vinyasa* has an equivalent breath: an inhale, an exhale, or a hold. A good general guideline is to exhale when going into forward bends and inhale when going into backbends.

The right breathwork in a *vinyasa* can make or break the success of a series. Before you begin your *vinyasa*, determine your pace and your intention. For instance, maybe you decide to do the sun salutation in a slow and languid way this morning, to warm you up. Let your breathing reflect this intention. Inhale and exhale deeply with each movement of this *vinyasa*. Then, this afternoon, perhaps you do it again, but this time at a quicker, more energized pace. Again, let your breathing reflect your intention. Breathe to the rhythm of your movements so your breath and your body work together.

Let your mind work with your body, using your breath as a monitor. If you can't breathe slowly enough, deepen your breath or allow for more than one breath in a position. If you can't keep up, slow the pace. Let your breath work for you. It will tell you when you are pushing yourself too hard.

Always remember to breathe with your entire body during *vinyasa*. Inhale fully, exhale completely. Let the movements, the contractions and expansions, the bends and arches, twists and stretches help your lungs and the muscles in your thoracic cavity to draw breath in and push it out. Feel the breath traveling from your toes to your fingertips, your heels to your head. Let the breath be as integral to the movement as your physical body.

Wise Yogi Tells Us

When you set your intention ahead of time, you'll be in a better frame of mind to notice and monitor your progress as you go. Are you revving up too much, when you had intended to go slow? Are you lagging behind when you had intended to keep an upbeat pace?

Body/Mind in Motion

Just as your breath works for you during *vinyasa*, so does your mind. More than your muscles are moving here! Your mind can and should be equally engaged in the movement from yoga pose to yoga pose.

Making a purposeful effort to concentrate on the way your body feels and moves during *vinyasa* is an excellent way to cultivate mindfulness. *Vinyasa* becomes a sort of meditation when practiced with this kind of intense focus. Let your moving body and flowing breath be the center of your meditation. Observe yourself from the inside out. Let your mind become the movement, let the movement become your body, let your body connect back to your mind in a complete circle.

You are one fully integrated, fully functioning *yogi*—so let's go with the flow!

Uttanatavasan: Leg Lifts

Uttanatavasan (pronounced *ooh-TAHN-ah-tah-VAH-sahn*), leg lifts, involve a steady-pose. They prepare the body to make the more fluid movements of a *vinyasa*. Leg lifts strengthen your stomach, which in turn supports your lower back. The deeper your breathing during this movement, the easier and smoother your *vinyasa* will become. Leg lifts also help prepare your body for a headstand. (Remember the headstand in Chapter 15, "Come on, Body, Let's Do the Twist"?)

Be careful not to let momentum swing your legs up during leg lifts. Keep your movements slow and complete to build your strength, touching the ground and pausing before each lift. Don't separate your feet or bend your knees when you come down. If your back hurts, keep one knee bent, foot on the floor, but keep the other leg straight.

If you have a sensitive back, bend the knee you are not lifting and keep that foot firmly on the ground. This will protect your lower back as you continue to strengthen it with leg lifts. Leg lifts build stomach and back muscles.

A Yoga Minute

Continuous practice of leg lifts can help alleviate lower back pain. A majority of Americans over 40 suffer from it.

A single leg lift.

1. Lie on your back. Bend your left leg slightly and press your lower back toward the floor slightly to avoid lower-back strain.

2. Inhale as you straighten your right leg and lift it straight up to the sky. When your leg is perpendicular to the floor, push your heel out.

3. Exhale and slowly lower your leg back down.

4. Repeat this movement on the same side, connecting each repetition with breath: Inhale as your leg goes up, exhale as your leg goes down.

5. After a satisfying number of repetitions (three or four, more if you are up for it), switch to your left leg.

And now for the double leg lift.

1. Begin the double leg lift with your palms facing down and tucked under your tailbone to keep your lower back from rising off the floor. Straighten your arms out underneath you. If you have long arms they may go past the tailbone, which is fine.

2. Slowly inhale as you bring both legs straight up while you contract your abdominal muscles, pulling them in toward the floor to further support your lower back.

3. Exhale as you bring both legs straight down, keeping your abdominals firmly contracted.

4. Do as many lifts as you can, inhaling as your leg goes up, exhaling as your leg goes down. Then rest.

Wise Yogi Tells Us

While flowing through a leg lift, cup your hands over your ears and listen intently to your breath as it connects movement to movement. Is it smooth? Rocky? Does it sound like the ocean? The wind in the trees? Link the rhythm of your breath to the movements of your muscles. Notice everything. Be mindful. Look inward.

Surya Namaskara: Sun Salutation

The sun is the center of our solar system, and without its energy and warmth, we wouldn't be able to exist on this planet. This *vinyasa* is a devotional (not to mention great exercise). *Surya namaskara* (pronounced *SOOR-yah nah-mahs-KAH-rah*) offers thanks and greetings to the sun, and although it can be performed any time, it is particularly appropriate and wonderful when performed at sunrise, out-of-doors, facing east. *Surya* means "sun," and *namaskara* literally means "taking a bow."

The sun salutation energizes, strengthens, and tones all the major muscles and organs in the body.

Chandra Namaskara: Moon Salutation

This *vinyasa* restores vitality, strength, and flexibility to the entire body. It also improves digestion through the continual compression of the intestinal tract. *Chandra* means "moon," and just as the sun salutation greets and honors the sun, so *chandra-namaskara* (pronounced *SHAHN-drah-nah-MAHS-kah-rah*) greets and honors the moon. Try practicing this *vinyasa* outside on a clear evening when the moon is in full view. Serenity!

Quite an energetic sequence of poses! The moon is a lunar/emotional/yin symbol. The strong physical movements in a moon salutation help to balance our emotional side with our physical side.

Ouch!

When performing the sun salutation, keep your awareness focused. If you go too fast, your mind may stray from attending to the body, breath, and devotion to the sun. You should go fast enough to keep the movements flowing and get your body warm, but not so fast that you don't feel in control of your movements or breath.

Know Your Sanskrit

Namaste (pronounced *nah–MAHS–tay*) is a **mudra** (hand position) in which the palms and fingers come together in the prayer position. Hands are held with your thumbs against the chest in an attitude of focused devotion. *Namaste* can also be held loosely behind the back with the fingers pointed up. *Namaste* means "Obeisance to you" or "I salute the divine light within you."

1. Begin in the mountain pose with your hands in *namaste,* or prayer position. Center yourself and concentrate on a devotional attitude.

2. Inhale. Raise your arms up over your head and tilt them slightly back, as if you were encompassing the sun with love.

3. Exhale. Bring your hands straight down to the floor. Bend your knees to protect your lower back. Eventually, you may straighten your legs. Bring your palms alongside your feet. This position is a symbol of thanking the earth, where our feet are firmly planted.

4. Keeping your hands down, inhale and step your right foot back behind you. Stay low to the ground and look up. This represents that we are on the earth through the strength of the sun.

5. Exhale. Bring both legs back behind you and balance in the plank pose, as if you were about to lower yourself into a pushup. Push out at the heels for strength. This represents finding a balance between the sun and the earth. Pause.

6. Exhale further. Bring your knees, chest, and chin to the floor. Keep your tailbone up off the ground. You are thanking the earth.

7. Inhale into the upward facing dog pose and look up. Let the sun's warmth strengthen you.

8. Exhale and push up into the downward facing dog pose, lengthening your spine. Let the strength of the sun enter your spine.

9. Inhale as you bring your right foot forward. Look up and thank the sun as you proceed on your journey.

10. Exhale and bring both legs together. With your palms alongside your feet, humbly devote yourself to the sun. Open your moon *chakra* (located at the back of your head) to the sun's kind and steady energy.

11. Inhale as you bring your arms and body up, tilting into a slight backbend, again embracing the sun with love.

12. Exhale as you bring your hands back into the prayer position, standing in *tadasana*, the mountain pose.

13. Repeat the entire sequence again for a complete round. For the second half-round, bring your left leg back first to create a balance.

1. Stand in the mountain pose with hands in *namaste,* or the prayer position. Inhale and bring your arms over your head in a slight backbend, keeping your palms together. You are greeting the moon.

2. Exhale and bring your palms to the floor. You are thanking the earth for allowing you to stand on it.

3. Inhale and step your left foot back. Touch the side of your ankle to the floor. Your right leg is lunged forward with the weight of your body on your toes.

4. Exhale and switch the position of your feet. Keep your left knee at a right angle to the floor with your right knee touching the floor. Your weight is now supported by your left foot and right knee. Inhale and lift your arms straight up overhead toward the moon.

5. Then exhale into the child's pose (see Chapter 18), a symbol of turning inward.

6. Now inhale and step your right foot back with the side of your ankle touching the floor. Your left leg is lunged forward with the weight of your body on your toes. Exhale and switch the position of your feet as before. Your right knee is at a right angle to the floor and your left knee is touching the floor. Your weight is now supported by your right foot and left knee.

7. Inhale and lift your arms straight up overhead. Thank you, moon!

8. Then exhale and bring your hands back to the floor. Inhale into the upward facing dog pose. Strong and steady, the moon circles us.

9. Exhale into the child's pose again—the moon *chakra* at the back of your head will open for healing energy.

10. Inhale, bring your hands straight up overhead, and look up.

11. Exhale and bring your hands back to the floor. Inhale, push your hands against the floor, and stand up into the mountain pose.

12. *Namaste.*

Create Your Own Flow

The sun and moon salutations are popular *vinyasa* because they combine a series of poses that so nicely balance each other (a backbend, then a forward bend, and so on). But you, too, can create your own series of postures. Just keep them balanced— forward with backward, exhale with inhale, upright with inverted, one side with the other side, an expansion with a contraction, and so on. This will become easier as you familiarize yourself with the postures in this book.

Here are a few suggestions to get you started. All poses mentioned here are described elsewhere in this book or are explained here.

Warm Wonder Vinyasa

Starting in the downward facing dog (Chapter 18, "Take the Forward Path"), flow into the plank pose (Chapter 13, "What Do You Stand For?"), which is like a pushup pose with the arms straight. Exhale, bend the elbows, and lower the body straight to the floor. Inhale, push yourself up into the upward facing dog (Chapter 14, "Bending

189

Over Backbends"), exhale, push back into the downward facing dog, inhale, push one leg forward, turn to the side, and straighten up into the triangle pose (Chapter 13). Do both sides in the triangle, then exhale as you bend your other knee and bring your hands alongside your foot. Push back into the downward facing dog. Hold for as long as comfortable, exhale into the child's pose (Chapter 18), then rest.

Solar Flare Vinyasa

Start in the mountain pose (Chapter 13), then jump your feet three to four feet apart and assume the warrior 2 pose (Chapter 13). Hold for a few breaths, then change your body position to face forward with your arms overhead in the warrior 1 pose (Chapter 13). Hold for a few breaths. Switch to the other side, doing warrior 1 and 2 in the other direction. Now, keeping your feet separated, turn your entire body to face forward and bend straight over with your knees straight. Bring your hands to-ward the floor and hold for a few breaths. Come back up, jump your feet together, bend your knees, and place your palms flat on the floor. Bend down into the child's pose (Chapter 18). Rest.

Mild and Mindful Vinyasa

Start in *shavasana* (Chapter 19, "Dead to the World"). Inhale and bring your hands under your tailbone, lifting up into the half fish pose (Chapter 14). Hold for a few breaths, then come out of the pose, exhaling, and rolling over into the child's pose (Chapter 18). Stay in the child's pose for a few breaths, inhale, sit up, exhale, and move into the hero pose (Chapter 17). Inhale as you move up, then exhale into the staff pose (Chapter 17). Inhale into any meditation pose (take your pick—see Chapter 17), and—you guessed it! Meditate for a while.

Moving with the Universe

While many yoga poses imitate animals or structures in nature (mountains, trees, and so on), *vinyasa* imitates the rhythm and movement of the natural world, the uni-verse, the cosmos. The human body is like a universe in microcosm, with its own in-ternal rhythms and movements. At the atomic level, the very atoms that make up everything are like tiny universes. Beyond our bodies, the world is full of cycles: the seasons, the years, the moons spinning around the planets, the planets spinning around the sun, the entire galaxy revolving.

Vinyasa helps us to feel a part of this magnificent, intricate, ultimately large and ulti-mately small cycle. The sun and the moon and the earth all move in concert, and through *vinyasa* we move in concert, too. Everything is moving to a sacred rhythm, ancient and eternal, and the rhythm wouldn't be the same if any one thing did not move with it. We are all part of a wave in the ocean of the universe, and when we move with the tide, we are doing what comes naturally, what makes us a part of the whole.

Now if that's not a good reason to do *vinyasa* every day, we don't know what is!

The Least You Need to Know

➤ A *vinyasa*, such as the sun or moon salutation, is a sequence of postures strung together and performed in a series of flowing movements.

➤ A *vinyasa* is coordinated with the breath and the mind so that body, breath, and mind are integrated.

➤ The sun salutation is the most well-known *vinyasa*, but many others exist, and you can even create your own by doing sequences of poses that balance each other.

➤ *Vinyasas* are great exercise for body and soul!

Part 5

Calming Down: Postures to Quiet the Body and Mind

These postures balance those in Part 4, calming and quieting the body and mind. First are the sitting poses in Chapter 17, "Are You Sitting Down?" including poses excellent for meditation. Sitting poses center the body and are conducive to a calm and tranquil mind.

Forward-bending poses are internalizing. As the body bends forward, folding in on itself, the mind can focus more easily inward. Chapter 18, "Take the Forward Path," describes forward bends, both sitting and standing, for you to try.

Chapter 19, "Dead to the World," is devoted to the most important of all the postures: shavasana. Also known as the corpse pose, shavasana is both the easiest and most difficult, because it involves simply lying on the floor in an attitude of complete and total relaxation. Sound easy? Just wait until you try to clear that active mind and keep that restless body still! Ten minutes of shavasana every day is a great way to manage the stresses in your life.

Chapter 17

Are You Sitting Down?

In This Chapter

➤ The sitting postures: staff, butterfly, hero, and cow

➤ Special poses for meditation: easy and kneeling

➤ Finally, the lotus pose!

It's time to take a load off! Lots of great and challenging yoga postures, as well as the meditative postures, are accomplished while sitting. Sitting poses keep your hips and legs flexible. You may even want to adapt some of the following poses for when you happen to be sitting on the floor outside of your regular yoga practice—just one more way to fit yoga into your day!

Flooring It

Everybody turf it! Yes, sit down on the floor. (Perhaps a welcome relief after a strenuous round of sun salutations.) You should feel comfortable in sitting poses, especially the meditative poses, because your body shouldn't distract you from your meditation. If you have a hard floor, a yoga mat or rug (one that won't slide around) will keep you comfortable. A carpeted floor is also fine. Don't use your bed—your practice surface should be comfortable but firm. You'll need the resistance of the floor for many of the postures, and a bed has too much "give." Ready? Set? Sit!

Dandasana: Staff Pose

A staff is a big stick used for support, like a walking stick. It is also a symbol of authority—he or she who holds the staff has the appearance of being large and in charge! Staff pose helps us to internalize this feeling of confidence, increasing our concentration and clarity of focus. *Dandasana* (pronounced *dahn-DAH-sah-nah*) is also great for your alignment. Concentrate on your upper body becoming straight and powerful as a staff.

The staff pose.

1. Sit on the floor with your feet straight out in front of you. Keep your palms flat alongside your hips with your fingers pointing toward your feet. Keep your knees and toes together, your heels pushed out, your toes relaxed. Your shoulders should be down, your chest open.

2. Push your palms lightly down against the ground to create space in your spine. Lengthen the top and bottom of your body. Center your weight over your hips. Breathe.

If the staff pose is uncomfortable, sit on a folded blanket until you become more flexible. Don't puff out your chest. Imagine, instead, that your head is being pulled upward, which will also keep your back from sinking down and your chin from coming up. Your chin should be in line with the floor.

Baddha Konasana: Butterfly Pose

Literally translated as "bound angle pose," this pose imitates a butterfly resting its wings on a lotus blossom. When holding *baddha konasana* (pronounced *BAH-dah koh-NAH-sah-nah*), imagine the delicate beauty of this image of the butterfly. The butterfly pose opens your hips and Jupiter *chakra* (the *chakra* located in your pelvic area; see Chapter 20, "*Chakras, Mudras, Mantras,* and *Mandalas*"). It also loosens your knees and ankles.

The butterfly pose.

1. Sit on the floor and bring the soles of your feet together, drawing them toward your body.

2. Open your chest and press your knees toward the ground as far as they will go. Don't bounce your legs up and down. Instead, allow gravity to gently release your hip joints.

3. Tilt your lower back inward to align the spine. Don't let your lower back sway out.

4. As your hips loosen, you will eventually be able to bow forward.

5. **Getting Started:** Some people find the butterfly pose easy because they have naturally loose hip joints. For others whose hips are less flexible, this pose can be frustrating. If you fall into the less-flexible category, place a pillow under each knee. Press your knees into the pillows, rather than all the way down to the floor. The more you do this pose, the more hip flexibility you will gain.

197

Wise Yogi Tells Us

While practicing the butterfly, keep your entire back straight. If your upper back becomes rounded as you pull your feet in, leave your feet farther from your body; hold on to your shins or thighs if you can't reach your feet. Concentrate on the image of the butterfly. If you catch yourself frowning with unpleasant effort, loosen the pose a bit, think about beauty, and smile!

Virasana: **Be a Hero!**

A hero stands tall and proud, even when sitting on the floor! The hero pose refreshes your legs, stretches your knees, and balances your Saturn *chakra* (located at the base of your spine). *Virasana* is pronounced *vir-AH-sah-nah.*

The hero pose also teaches you to expand your breathing space even while sitting. Imagine lifting from the top of your head and anchoring your hips to the floor. Let your breath expand everything in between.

Feel your breath while sitting in the hero pose.

The hero pose can be hard on delicate knees if performed too quickly or attempted before your flexibility allows it. Go very gradually into this pose so you can feel at what point your knees are telling you to stop. If this is hard to do, sit on a telephone book. Every time you practice, tear out one page. In other words, go slow. You'll get a little farther each time.

The hero pose.

1. Breathe deeply ... heroes *always* breathe deeply. (That's how they stay calm in the face of adversity!) Feel your diaphragm lowering as your body fills with air.

2. Sit back on your heels, gradually separating your feet until you are sitting on the floor between your legs.

3. Keep your knees from buckling in, and move your lower back forward without inflating your upper chest.

Gomukhasana: Holy Cow!

To us Westerners, the cow may be less than glamorous. Sure, it may adorn the pot holders, aprons, and cookie jars in our country kitchens, and we may think cows are awfully cute, but we don't take them too seriously. In India, however, the

Ouch!

Don't be frustrated if your hands can't grasp each other. You don't want to pull a muscle! Have the patience of a cow. You'll get there eventually. Cows take their sweet time, and so should you!

199

cow is the most sacred of animals, worshipped for its giving nature—cream, butter, and dung, which is used as fuel for fire. Appropriately, the cow pose is meant to lead to a feeling of openness and giving. It also stimulates the nerves at the base of your spine, aids in longevity as it keeps your lower vertebrae from calcifying, opens your shoulders and chest, and activates your Saturn and Jupiter *chakras* (located at the base of your spine and in your pelvic area, respectively), helping to raise *kundalini* energy. *Gomukhasana* (pronounced *goh-moo-KHA-sah-nah*) is composed of *go*, which means "cow," *mukha*, which means "mouth" or "face," and of course, *asana*, which means "posture."

The cow pose.

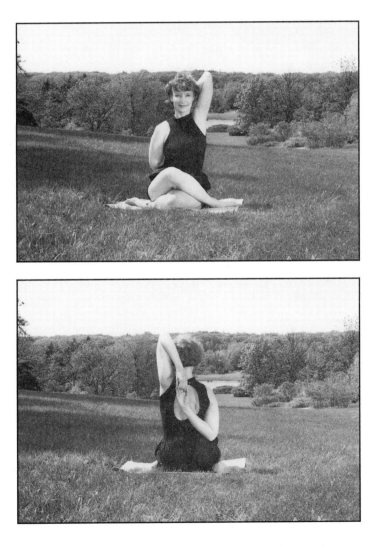

1. Sit with your legs in front of you, then bring one knee on top of the other. Draw your heels toward your body in this cross-legged position.

2. Point one elbow toward the sky, with your palm facing back behind you. Point the other elbow toward the ground, with your palm facing out behind you. Bring your hands toward each other, clasping them if you can.

Meditative Poses

Technically, you can meditate just about anywhere and in any position, but ideally, you should try to meditate in one of several meditative poses. Why? There's nothing magical about the meditative poses, except that they arrange your body in a way ideal for meditation. Your spine is aligned so energy can flow freely. Your body is relaxed and comfortable. Meditative poses should feel so wonderful that you barely notice your body. If a meditative pose is uncomfortable or painful, you aren't quite ready for it yet. Try a different one.

Mudras are special hand positions you can use while meditating to channel energy back through the fingers into the spinal column's *chakras*, directing and rebalancing *prana* in the body. Choose from the *mudras* in the following illustration; mix and match *mudras* to enhance your yoga practice of meditation. (See Chapter 20 for more on *chakras* and *mudras*.)

A Yoga Minute

People who meditate are less sensitive to carbon dioxide.

Wise Yogi Tells Us

Placing your hands with the palms down on your knees gives you a sense of grounding and centering energy. Placing your hands with the palms up on your knees gives you a sense of releasing energy, opening, and liberation.

Mudras *for meditation.*

Namaste

OM

Jnana

Buddhi

Sukhasana: *Easy Pose*

Sukhasana (pronounced *soo-KAH-sah-nah*) is a great meditation pose for be-ginners. *Sukha* means "joy," and this pose should feel so good that it fills you with joy! *Sukhasana* facilitates *pranayama*, quiets the mind, and stills the body.

The easy pose.

1. Sit in a simple crossed-leg position, with either leg on top. Try to sit more often with the leg that is least comfortable on top, to balance your body. Rest your

hands on your knees and breathe. Do not be concerned if your knees do not yet rest on the ground. This will come in time as the hips open.

2. If your back starts to arch, put a pillow under your tailbone to align the spine. Think about happiness and joy!

Vajrasana: *Kneeling Pose*

Vajrasana (pronounced *vahj-RAH-sah-nah*) is also called the Zen pose, as this is the meditation pose used by *Zen Buddhist* monks. *Vajra* means "thunderbolt" or "diamond." *Vajrasana* aids circulation to the feet, lifts the spinal column, and relieves pressure on the diaphragm.

The kneeling pose.

A Yoga Minute

Zen is a sect of Buddhism in which enlightenment is sought through sitting meditation or contemplating enigmatic riddles called *koans*, rather than through the formal study of religious texts. **Buddhism** is a religion with many sects that teaches right living, right thinking, and meditation as a means to enlightenment. For more on Zen, look for *The Complete Idiot's Guide to Zen Living*, by Gary McClain, Ph.D., and Eve Adamson.

1. Again, breathe! Sit back on your heels, keeping your heels and knees together.

2. Keeping your spine straight, place your hands on your knees. If your knees hurt, go back to the easy pose, and smile! If they don't hurt, enjoy *this* pose, and smile!

Padmasana: *Lotus Pose*

At last, the venerable lotus pose! You've heard about it, maybe you've seen it, perhaps you've even tried it. *Padmasana* (pronounced *pahd-MAH-sah-nah*) represents a lotus flower open to the light (*padma* means "lotus"). It keeps the spine from sagging and keeps you comfortable in meditation for longer periods of time than other positions. It also keeps your body from toppling over if you fall asleep during meditation (many wise souls have!). The lotus position keeps your chest open, gives your diaphragm lots of room, and opens your Venus *chakra* (located behind your heart).

The lotus flower is considered sacred because it is beautiful, symmetrical, and has a long root that reaches down into the depths of a pond. The lotus flower has its roots in the muddy earth, but it works its way through the mud and eventually blooms into a perfect white flower facing the heavens!

It's easy to be so concerned with trying to achieve the lotus pose that you forget the point of being in the pose: to be comfortable in your body. Because yoga is such an internal process, even if you're sitting in a perfect lotus pose in what appears to be quiet meditation, inside you may not be practicing yoga at all. You may be distracted, worried, or suffering. You might be stuck in the mud! True meditation is joyful.

If your ankles or any other part of you (including your feelings) is in agony or pain, meditation will be much more difficult to achieve. Find an easier pose, or postpone meditation in favor of more active postures. (Exercise is great when you're feeling low.) Come back to meditation when your mind is ready—and only then—in a position your body loves.

The lotus pose.

1. Sit on the floor and begin to breathe deeply.

2. Place your left ankle on top of your right thigh so the sole of your foot faces upward. Then move your right ankle to the top of your left thigh so the sole of your other foot faces upward (or the other way around—and next time, try to switch which foot is on top).

3. Shift a little to center your weight on your hip bones, then place your hands, palms up or down, on your knees. This pose should feel very stable.

4. Ideally, your body will form a tripod, with both knees and your body touching the ground. If you can't get your knees down toward the ground, you can sit on a cushion or pillow. This can also make the pose easier for people with less-flexible hips.

Ouch!

If your ankles, hips, or knees begin to hurt, practice nonviolence by returning to the easy pose. The lotus pose requires strong ankles and open hips. Practice yoga's standing postures to build ankle and hip strength.

Baddha Padmasana: *Bound Lotus Pose*

The bound lotus is the same as the lotus, except that your right arm goes behind your back and holds your right foot, while your left arm goes behind your back and holds your left foot. This pose is even more stable and symmetrical than the lotus pose. Whichever arm crosses on top, go the opposite way next time. *Baddha padmasana* (pronounced *BAH-dah pahd-MAH-sah-nah*) deepens all the benefits of the lotus pose, and you'll be able to breathe more deeply. This is considered a more advanced pose than the advanced lotus pose. Butterfly pose (described earlier in this chapter) is an excellent warm-up pose to create the hip flexibility needed for stability in regular and bound lotus poses.

The bound lotus pose.

The Least You Need to Know

➤ Sitting postures strengthen and increase flexibility in your hips and legs.

➤ *Mudras* are hand positions that enhance meditation by rechanneling energy that emanates from the fingers back into the body where it can stimulate the *chakras*.

➤ Meditate only in a posture that is perfectly comfortable. Some suggestions: easy, kneeling, and lotus.

➤ A straight spine makes a meditation pose meditative.

➤ If you're down, move around. Feeling great? Meditate!

Chapter 18

Take the Forward Path

In This Chapter

➤ Why bend forward?

➤ Forward bends: child's pose, standing head to knees, feet apart side angle, sitting one leg, bound half lotus, *yoga mudra*, boat, tortoise, and downward facing dog

➤ Modifications, challenges, and other tips to improve your yoga practice

---

Forward bends are important for several reasons. They're wonderful for helping you to focus inward and quiet your mind. As your body bends forward, it folds your heart into its center. Forward bends are also important to balance backbends, so include a few of each in your yoga practice.

Forward bends are great for stretching out and loosening up the lower back muscles and also for lengthening the hamstrings. Believe it or not, the leg muscles often hold more stress than any other muscle group in the body! Forward bends help you reach that inner place where you can allow the lower back and hamstrings to relax and become fluid. Okay … one, two, three, reach!

Mudhasana: Child's Pose

The child's pose makes you feel safe and nurtured, as if you were still in the womb. *Mudhasana* (pronounced *moo-DAH-sah-nah*) activates your Venus and moon *chakras* (located behind your heart and at the base of your skull, respectively), relieves lower back pain, and improves your complexion. It also stimulates respiration because it compresses your diaphragm.

When practicing the child's pose, put some pillows or a blanket under your head to help lengthen your back if you find it hard to bend forward, or place a pillow or blanket between your knees and calves if your knees feel strained.

The child's pose.

1. Sit back on your heels, then bring your forehead to the floor.

2. Rest your arms alongside your body with your palms facing up. The pose should feel completely relaxing.

3. Breathe deeply. Feel your diaphragm rising and sinking with each breath, like a baby's tummy. A baby hasn't yet learned shallow chest-breathing.

Uttanasana: **Standing Head to Knees Pose**

Uttanasana (pronounced *OOH-tah-NAH-sah-nah*) stretches the entire back of your body. It also tones your abdomen, decreases bloating, refreshes your mind, and clears your head. To accomplish this, you may have to bend your knees. As you become more flexible, you'll be able to grasp your big toes with your index fingers. For those who can fold in half, give yourselves a hug!

1. Stand with your feet together. Inhale and raise your arms overhead.

2. Exhale and bend forward at your hips. Bending at the waist will curve your back. Try to bend at the hip joint to keep the heart open as you move forward. Work toward touching your nose to your knees. Keep your knees straight unless your back hurts, in which case you can bend your knees.

3. Be careful not to rock your weight back to your heels. Keep your weight evenly distributed over your feet. Don't round your back or turn your feet out; instead,

bend forward from the hips, lengthening through the lower back. Don't force your head toward your knees—let gravity do the work as your head and neck stay relaxed. Don't be concerned with how far you bend. Focus on how open you can become as you "lift" forward.

The standing head to knees pose.

Parshvottanasana: Feet Apart Side Angle Pose

In *parshvottanasana* (pronounced *PARSH-voh-tah-NAH-sah-nah*), you will tone your abdomen; straighten drooping shoulders; and make your hips, spine, and wrists more flexible.

The feet apart side angle pose.

1. Stand with your feet three to four feet apart. Turn one foot out and face that foot.

2. Bring your hands into the *namaste* or prayer position, but behind your back with your fingers pointing up. If this is too difficult, simply clasp your hands behind your back, or keep your hands at your sides as you move forward.

3. Inhale, lengthen the spine upward, then exhale, bringing your head toward your front knee.

4. Imagine your chest, rather than your head, moving toward your knees to help lengthen the spine and prevent rounding of the back. Keep breathing throughout this pose.

Janu Shirshasana: Sitting One Leg Pose

In *janu shirshasana* (pronounced *JAH-noo shur-SHAH-sah-nah*), *janu* means "knee," and *shirsha* means "head." You may guess that this pose, then, involves bringing the head and knee together. The sitting one leg pose tones your abdomen, liver, spleen, and kidneys. It quiets your mind and aids digestion, as well as stretches and strengthens your lower back and chest. Men suffering from an enlarged prostate will benefit from this pose.

The sitting one leg pose.

210

1. Sit on the floor with your left leg straight in front of you, toes pointed up. Your right leg should be bent in toward the straight leg.

2. Raise your hands over your head, exhale, and slowly bend forward over your straight leg.

3. Hold the stretch, then inhale as you rise back up. Repeat on the other side.

4. **Yoga Adventure:** As you become more flexible, you'll be able to grasp your foot with your hands. Maybe not today, but that's okay!

Wise Yogi Tells Us

If you feel stress on your back doing the sitting one leg pose, bend the knee you are reaching toward. Angle your body directly over this knee. Release any competitive thoughts. Forget your goals and open your heart. Bend at the hips, not at the waist. Don't hurry, smile, and be patient with yourself. Slowly your leg and hip will open. Have fun with the process.

Ardha Baddha Padma Pashchimottanasana: Bound Half Lotus Pose

Ardha baddha padma pashchimottanasana (pronounced *AHR-dah BAH-dah PAHD-mah PAH-shih-moh-tah-NAH-sah-nah*) is identical to the sitting one leg pose, except that the foot of your bent leg is in a half lotus position, with one foot placed on the opposite thigh.

Ouch!

Not every pose is for every body. Be patient and kind with your body, and your body will respond accordingly. You will be amazed at the power of TLC (tender loving care!).

1. Sit on the floor with one leg in front of you (as in the sitting one leg pose) and the other leg bent, foot placed on your opposite thigh in the half lotus.

2. Bring your arm around your back and connect your hand to this foot.

211

3. Face your upper torso directly over your extended leg. Open your chest, exhale, and slowly bend forward. Repeat on the other side. If you can't achieve this pose, be patient and don't push your body. The pose will come.

The bound half lotus pose.

Wise Yogi Tells Us

Just a friendly reminder to your ego: Take a hike! When performing any yoga pose, especially more difficult poses, don't allow your ego to take over. If you find yourself thinking, "Look at me touching the floor!" or "Wow, I'm so good at this!" re-adjust your thoughts. The goal of yoga is to eliminate ego, not to encourage it. Feel how the posture you're holding helps your mind to become clear and see the truth: that you are one with the true world.

Yoga Mudra: Ego-Be-Gone!

Yoga mudra (pronounced *YOH-gah MOO-drah*) is a symbol of unity. This important pose inspires feelings of devotion and humility. It also stretches your legs and hips, opens your shoulders, and aids the gastrointestinal tract.

The yoga mudra *pose.*

1. Sit cross-legged or in the kneeling pose.

2. Move your arms behind your back, clasp your hands, and lower your head to the floor.

3. Keeping your arms straight, lift your clasped hands up over your head until your arms are perpendicular to the floor.

4. **Yoga Adventure:** Bring your hands into *namaste* (remember the *namaste mudra* from Chapter 17, "Are You Sitting Down?") and let them rest on your middle back.

Naukasana: Boat Pose

A *yogi* holding *naukasana* (pronounced *now-KAH-sah-nah*) looks like a boat bobbing on the waves, and *nauka* literally means "ship." This pose tones your stomach and intestines, strengthens your back, and activates your Mars *chakra* (located behind your navel).

In the boat pose, don't hold your breath, even as you are concentrating on balancing. Your feet may fall to the floor at first. Whether you are doing the full boat pose or the half boat pose (see the following description), keep your leg position steady and your knees together.

The boat pose.

1. For the full boat pose, sit on the floor with your knees bent in front of you and your arms holding your knees.

2. Lean back to about a 45-degree angle, bring your feet off the floor, and balance on your tailbone.

3. Raise your feet straight up in the air so your body forms a V shape. For balance, extend your arms straight out, parallel to the floor at about knee level.

4. Imagine you are bobbing on top of the water like a little rowboat.

The half boat pose.

5. **Getting Started:** If balancing in the full boat pose is too difficult at first, start with the half boat pose. Keep your knees bent, but instead of raising your feet all the way up raise them to a right angle to the floor. Keep your knees together. Bring your hands alongside your feet with your palms facing in.

Kurmasana: **Tortoise Pose**

You'll look like a tortoise when you practice *kurmasana* (pronounced *koohr-MAH-sah-nah*). This pose keeps your lumbar limber! (In other words, it makes your lower spine more flexible.) It also strengthens your neck, massages your thyroid, aids digestion, and rejuvenates your nervous system. Take it slow—just like a tortoise!

Does the tortoise pose seem impossible? Simply lower yourself as far as you can, smile, and enjoy the journey to the floor, even if it takes many, many yoga practices. Tortoises are not in a hurry. They live looooong lives!

A Yoga Minute

Hypothyroidism, the underproduction of the thyroid hormone, is a common condition and may be the underlying cause of many recurring illnesses and chronic fatigue. Symptoms of an underactive thyroid include fatigue, weight gain, weakness, dry skin, hair loss, recurrent infections, depression, and intolerance to cold.

The tortoise pose.

1. Sit with your legs extended in front of you in a V shape. Bend your knees just slightly, and slide your arms under your knees with your palms on the floor.

2. Slowly straighten your legs again to hold your arms against the floor, and bring your chest forward. Your chin will eventually reach the floor.

Adho Mukha Shvanasana: **Downward Facing Dog Pose**

Another pose named after the esteemed canine. Downward facing dog, *adho mukha shvanasana* (pronounced *AH-doh MOO-kah shvah-NAH-sah-nah*), brings heat to your body, strengthens and stretches your spine, and gives your heart a rest.

This is one of the better known yoga poses—maybe because it feels so great to do it! Downward facing dog is easily adjustable for any flexibility level. You can reach down to the floor, or even to the seat of a firmly anchored chair, if you can't quite make it all the way down. Or if you are very flexible, you can press all the way down to the floor with your palms and your heels while pushing your hips up. Ahh, doesn't that feel great?

If you have trouble with this pose because of tight hamstrings, spend extra yoga time on sitting forward bends to loosen the back of your legs. If downward facing dog hurts your wrists, you may not be balancing your weight evenly. Try to shift weight back into your heels. Hold the pose only as long as you are comfortable. Little by little, your balance will shift, and this pose will eventually become quite soothing.

Ouch!

If your back is sore or tight, definitely keep your knees bent. Focus on spine lengthening, not on your heels coming down.

It may also help to concentrate on stretching out your lower back. Instead of rounding it, lengthen it. Remember the way your back is stretched out in the child's pose? Think about lifting your tailbone to the sky. If necessary, keep your knees slightly bent to return a natural curve to your lower back. When you are flexible and strong enough to perform the downward facing dog fully and peacefully, you will place as much weight in your heels as you do in your hands. To get this feeling of the full pose, have a partner lift your hips up and shift your weight back to center, just as we show in the following illustration.

The downward facing dog pose.

1. Get down on your hands and knees. Lift your tailbone up, bringing your knees off the floor so your body forms an upside-down V, with your palms and the balls of your feet touching the floor.

2. Bring your head down and your hips up. Keep your knees bent at first, then slowly bring your heels to the floor and straighten your legs. Breathe and hold for as long as it feels good.

Feeling worn out yet? The next chapter will give you a chance to let your body really relax so all that work can take effect. The corpse pose is, paradoxically, the easiest and most challenging yoga pose of all. Read on to learn more, and prepare to get really, really relaxed.

The Least You Need to Know

➤ Forward-bending postures—such as standing head to knees, feet apart side angle, sitting one leg, bound half lotus, *yoga mudra,* boat, half boat, tortoise, and downward facing dog—help you to internalize and quiet your mind.

➤ Forward bends are great for loosening the lower back and stretching out the hamstrings.

➤ Forward bends and backbends balance each other and should be practiced together.

Chapter 19

Dead to the World

In This Chapter

➤ Why the corpse pose is so-named, and why it's the most important of all the poses

➤ More on *Om*

➤ How to relax and stop thinking

➤ Finding peace at last!

Of all the yoga poses, *shavasana* (pronounced *shah-VAH-sah-nah*), also known as the *corpse pose,* is the most important. *Shava* means "corpse," and just as it sounds, the corpse pose consists of lying on the floor in complete relaxation, still, peaceful, and corpse-like. "How can lying on the floor be important?" you might ask. Or better yet, "How can imitating a corpse be important?"

Both good questions! Here's a good answer: The essence of peace comes from within, not from without. *Shavasana*'s goal is to relax the body so completely that the body becomes irrelevant, as if it were deceased. With the body "gone," the mind is set free to blossom.

"But a corpse is dead!" you might continue to argue. "Isn't yoga about life?" Yes! But life and death are inseparable—they are all part of a bigger reality. By learning the corpse pose, you learn to live. By focusing inward, which means focusing beyond the body, the ego, and the superficial trappings of the "you" who walks around every day (clothes, habits, personality), you'll ultimately connect with the beauty of the universe. The surface "you" can finally fall away, and the inner "you," the Real You, can emerge. Imagine the resounding cosmic question: Will the Real You please stand up? If you've mastered *shavasana*, you'll know just who the Real You is! As your body lies corpse-like, the Real You can stand.

How to Be a Corpse

Shavasana involves more than collapsing onto the floor in a crumpled heap after a long, hard day and *wishing* you were dead. Let's practice the corpse pose with a little more focus!

Shavasana: *Yoga's corpse pose.*

1. Lie comfortably on your back on the floor, and separate your legs so your feet are two to three feet apart. Let your toes fall out to the sides. Close your eyes.

2. Separate your arms so that each hand is two to three feet from your body, with each palm facing up.

3. Roll your head from side to side, releasing tension in your neck.

4. Roll your shoulders down and away from your ears.

5. Allow your attention to travel up and down your body, scanning for tight spots or contracted muscles. When you find a tight spot, gently tell the area to relax (out loud, if it helps). For example, "Chill out, right shoulder!" You may have to say it twice. Place a pillow under your knees or head if this helps you relax.

6. Repeat your body scan until your body is completely relaxed.

7. Now bring your attention to your breath. Listen to your breath. Don't try to control it. Simply observe it. Feel it flowing in and out of you. Make the sound and feel of your breath the sole focus of your attention.

8. If part of your body starts to tense up, redirect your mind to the tense area and focus on relaxing it again. Then return to the breath.

9. As thoughts pop into your mind ("If my computer crashes again today, I'm gonna throw it out the window." "That new guy at the office sure is cute!"), let them pass back out of your mind. Imagine they are soap bubbles—allow your breath to blow them away softly, up into the sky.

10. Come back to the breath. Back to the breath. To the breath. The breath. Breath. *Om.*

One for All, and All for *Om!*

Maybe lying on the floor is no problem for you, but everything after that is a real challenge. It isn't easy to relax, let alone clear the mind. *Om* to the rescue! We've mentioned the *mantra Om* a few times already in this book, but let's look at it again in terms of its power to center and relax you. *Om* is the sound frequently chanted by *yogis,* because it is an all-encompassing sound. According to *yogic* thought, if all of life were translated into a single sound, the sound of the universe, that sound would be *Om.*

Try saying the sound now, right where you are sitting (or standing, or lying down, or wherever you happen to be at the moment). Take a deep breath, breathing from the diaphragm, and sing out the "O" sound as long as you can without your voice faltering. Don't be afraid to put some sound and strength behind it. If you're worried about keeping your volume down too much, you might not give the sound the breath support it requires. Stay strong and sing out the sound, which is pronounced like "OH," then slowly let the "O" sound come to a close in a resonating, vibrating "MMMMM" sound.

Now take a breath, close your eyes this time, and try it again. Let the sound stretch out for as long as you can with the support of a deep breath. Use up all your breath, but don't strain yourself. Doesn't that feel good? Do it again if you'd like to. Notice how, when your entire body is vibrating with that sound, it's easier to concentrate on the breath and the sound than whether to have dessert with dinner tonight or whether you can convince someone else to do the dishes.

A Yoga Minute

Gandhi's last words to his assailant as he fell to the ground, January 30, 1948, from a gunshot wound, were "Rama, Rama," which means "Praise God." This is the essence of yoga: to have one's thoughts continuously up-lifted, even (especially!) in the transition from one existence to another.

Also notice how much *Om* sounds like "amen." If you've been to or go to church, you've probably heard the "amen" sung at the end of every hymn. Have you ever noticed that when a chorus of voices sings "amen," the voices often bloom from a single note into a harmony, like a multipetaled flower opening in sound? Think how nicely this concept fits into the yoga way of thinking. Many voices harmonize to form a single, beautiful sound that is more complete than one voice alone, just as the universe is a beautiful blending of each soul into a single vibration of love.

In a nutshell, the point of chanting *Om* is to let the incredible power of sound and vibration work for you, pushing away worldly concerns and physical discomforts to bring your mind to a singular (yet universal) focus. Try it the next time you try the corpse pose. You'll be blissfully surprised!

When the Easiest Is the Hardest

Some of you may still be stuck on the idea that *shavasana* is the most important of all the postures. "How hard can it be?" you might wonder. "How hard can it be to lie on the floor and relax?" Actually, *shavasana* is also the most challenging pose, even though it seems, at first, to be the easiest. In a way, the corpse pose is both the easiest and the hardest pose. Unlike some poses, where you first need to spend a lot of time developing strong ankles or upper arms or balance, the corpse pose can be assumed by anyone who can lie on the floor.

On the other hand, not only is relaxation a true challenge for many, but *shavasana* has a strong mental component, without which you aren't truly practicing *shavasana*. Just as you can hold the lotus pose perfectly without truly practicing yoga, you can certainly lie in what appears to be a perfect *shavasana* without coming close to a *yogic*

Wise Yogi Tells Us

Even though *shavasana* isn't meant to put you to sleep, practicing it in bed at night—particularly the steps for relaxing the body—can help lure even the most hardcore insomniac toward dreamland.

state of mind. Ideally, *shavasana* could be practiced in the midst of total chaos, because the *yogi* in *shavasana* has utterly released him- or herself from the body. The body is merely a shell or a vessel, while the soul is directly connected with the universe. Certainly it takes a long while to reach this point, and the corpse pose can be practiced quite productively before this state is reached, but this is the ideal destination—and a challenging journey it is!

Let *shavasana* become a part of your workout, and take it just as seriously as any other posture—even *more* seriously. Your body will learn how to release all its tensions and will benefit even more from the other postures because of its time spent in *shavasana*. Your spirit, too, will learn how to soar beyond the limits of its "container." Now *that's* a powerful skill!

Open Up and Let Go: The Body

Your body is a complex organism with thousands of parts, all connected and related, yet separate, too. It's no easy task to relax the whole thing, let alone transcend it completely. When practicing *shavasana*, it can help to have a plan for releasing each part of your body a little at a time. Read over the following steps for releasing and relaxing the lower body, upper body, and face. Enough times through, and you'll have the steps memorized.

The Lower Body: Going Nowhere

Once you are in the corpse pose and have followed all the steps mentioned earlier, but before you focus on your breath, relax your lower body:

1. Tighten one foot, curling the toes and contracting your foot muscles for a few seconds. Then release and feel the tension flowing from your foot.

2. Flex your ankle and tighten your calf, then relax both.

3. Lift your entire leg two inches off the ground. Tense your leg, especially the large thigh muscle. Squeeze! Then let your leg fall to the ground. With the release, imagine all the tension falling away.

4. Repeat these three steps with your other foot and leg.

5. Lift your hips two inches off the floor and squeeze your buttocks as tightly as you can for several seconds. Then release the contraction and drop your hips back down. Feel all the tight areas releasing and relaxing. Your hip joints should feel loose and your buttocks muscles completely relaxed.

Ouch!

If lying flat on the floor is uncomfortable for your back, put pillows or blankets under your knees. This protects your lower back from undue strain. If your head or neck is uncomfortable, rest your head or neck on a small pillow, but make sure your throat feels open. Too many pillows could block the flow of energy through your neck; too few pillows could cause your neck to overstrain backward. If you have low blood pressure and your feet get cold, wear socks. Strive for a feeling of openness in all parts of your body.

The Upper Body: Still Rhythms

Continuing upward:

1. Contract your stomach muscles as tightly as you can, then release them.

2. Lift one arm about two inches off the floor. Squeeze your hand into a fist and hold it tightly. Flex your arm muscles for several seconds, then relax your entire arm and let it fall. Feel stress and tightness flowing down your arm and out the ends of your fingers. Repeat with the other arm.

3. Tighten your chest muscles, then release them. As you release them, try to feel your heartbeat. Gently tell your heart to relax, slow down, and rest.

4. Bring your shoulders up to your ears, tensing your shoulders for several seconds. Release them and feel all the stress dropping away. Many people carry tension in their shoulders. You may want to do this several times until your shoulders feel truly loose.

The Ultimate Facial: Losing Your Senses

And now for the rest of you:

1. Lift your head two inches off the ground. Tense all your neck and facial muscles, scrunching up your face like a prune. Purse your lips and imagine you are trying to bring every part of your face to your nose. Release and lower your head.

2. Raise your head again, and open your eyes and mouth as wide as you possibly can. Stick your tongue out as far as you can. Really stretch that face for several seconds, then relax and lower your head to the ground.

3. Roll your head slowly and gently from one side to the other.

4. One at a time, scan your senses. First, notice what you can taste, then let it go. Take your mind away from your taste buds. Next, notice what you can smell, then release your sense of smell. Notice everything your body is touching, then imagine you are floating and can't feel anything. What can you hear? Let it go. Turn off your ears and focus inward. Last of all, let go of your sight (even though your eyes should already be closed) by releasing all tension around your eyes. If you see light through your eyelids, gently push away your awareness of it.

5. Now go back over each body part again, but this time, instead of physically tensing and releasing your muscles, mentally tell each part to relax. Really focus on each area, one at a time, and coax it to release all pain and tension. Consider this the start of a wonderful relationship between your mind and your body. Why shouldn't they converse?

6. After you've completed all these steps, you should feel very, very relaxed and internalized. Mentally scan your body a few more times, seeking out pockets of stress and releasing them. If any sensations try to creep back in, gently ignore them.

Now you're ready to leave your body behind and ride the breath.

Open Up and Let Go: The Mind

You've moved past your body and are now immersed in your mind. But that has to go, too. Yes, the mind is as distracting as the body when it comes to true relaxation—maybe more so! Even as you lie in the corpse pose feeling proud that you've managed to transcend your body, at least to some extent, your mind is holding you back from true awareness. How? By making you feel proud, for one thing! Pride belongs to the ego, and in true awareness, there is no ego. So what's an active-minded person to do? Simple: Stop thinking.

Me? Stop Thinking? Forget About It!

To many, the prospect of not thinking seems far more of an effort than the most complicated yoga posture. We *are* our minds—aren't we? Not according to *yogic* philosophy. In fact, wise *yogis* tell us that we aren't our bodies or our minds at all. These are merely tools to help free our souls and bring them into fuller and more unifying consciousness.

As you rest in *shavasana* attempting to keep your mind at bay, think about your mind merely as a tool to help you in your task. When used at the wrong time or for the wrong job, a tool can be a hindrance, but when used correctly, it will make any job easier. During *shavasana*, it's time to put the tools down. Put away your thoughts. Let them go. You can always pick them up again later.

Dream a Little Dream

Imagine waking up one morning with the memory of a beautiful dream. In the dream, you are walking through your home, and everything is familiar until you come upon a door you've never noticed before. You open the door and step through it into a new universe. Pure beauty surrounds you, and you are filled with a sense of bliss. You realize that you are perfect. You have no faults, no sins, no shortcomings, no guilt. You are a being of pure light, and the whimsically lovely universe that encompasses you is also you. Love radiates from you and into you. You vaguely remember the comparatively ponderous and painful life of striving on the other side of the door through which you came, but as you look behind you, the door is gone, and you realize that other life was just a dream.

And then you wake up. Which was real, and which was the dream? *Yogic* philosophy says that this life we lead in these earthbound bodies and minds is the dream, and that pure bliss is the reality. Yoga helps us to wake from this dream. But even dreams exist for a reason, and we all move through this dream of our lives to learn about our souls. This dream is a lesson, but it's still only a dream (though an awfully vivid one!).

Of course, we don't mean that right now you are really asleep and dreaming all of this. Life isn't a dream in the sense that we are used to thinking of dreams. But according to wise *yogis*, our interpretation of life is an illusion. Anything that isn't eternal and blissful is an illusion. Yoga, and especially *shavasana*, helps us to work past our bodies and dig through our thoughts until we unearth the jewel that is cosmic consciousness. How extraordinary to awake to such a reality!

Ouch!

If your daily obligations make it impossible for you to get away for a restorative vacation, don't be discouraged. Practicing *shavasana* can give you the mental break you need.

Give Your Mind a Breather

But let's get back to this "dream" we're all living and striving through called life. We have to live in the world, and we can't lie in the corpse pose all day long. We have to eat, sleep, make money, do our daily chores, care for those who depend on us. What good is *shavasana* during the rest of the day?

Have you ever left all your worries behind and taken off for a vacation, even if just for the night? Maybe you found a last-minute baby-sitter and whisked your spouse off for a romantic evening alone. Maybe you took a personal day off from work, got in your car, and drove somewhere you'd never been before. If you've never done such a thing, you should try it. It's rejuvenating and gives you a new perspective on your everyday life. But even if you aren't at liberty to leave your regular life for a while, you can still practice *shavasana*—a mini-vacation for your mind.

Wise Yogi Tells Us

"Do not take life's experiences too seriously. Above all, do not let them hurt you, for in reality, they are nothing but dream experiences ... If circumstances are bad and you have to bear them, do not make them a part of yourself. Play your part in life, but never forget that it is only a role."

—Paramahansa Yogananda

If you had a job where you had to work the same hours your mind has to work, you'd probably collapse in less than a week. Of course, our brains are made to be busy, but even the most efficient brain needs a break now and then. *Shavasana* turns everything off: the senses, the emotions, the thoughts. Only breath exists, and pure consciousness. If you've ever uttered the words, "At last, I can just sit here and do nothing!" you know how your brain feels when you practice *shavasana*.

Quest for Peace

Perhaps the most compelling reason for us Westerners to practice *shavasana* is that it simply brings more peace into our lives. Imagine yourself calmer and more clear-headed, able to take any situation in stride, handle any emergency with unruffled confidence. The regular practice of *shavasana* can give you this gift. We can all use more peace in our lives, and this needn't be a futile wish. Take an active role in bringing peace to your life through *shavasana*, because even the most hectic and chaotic external life is miraculous and wonderful when peace lives inside you.

The Least You Need to Know

➤ If you practice only one yoga pose, practice *shavasana*.

➤ Mastering *shavasana* can be more strenuous and requires more discipline than the most physically demanding of yoga postures!

➤ In *shavasana*, first you consciously relax your body, then you consciously relax your mind, then you let your consciousness go, too, living only in the breath and pure awareness.

➤ Learning to quiet your mind and remove scattered thinking will bring you peace.

Part 6

Living Your Yoga

Part 6 will help you incorporate yoga into your daily life in lots of ways. First we go into more detail about chakras, mudras, mantras, *and* mandalas, *which can help you to refine, intensify, and optimize your yoga and meditation practice. Next we discuss diet and how what you eat can affect who you are. Yoga divides foods into three categories:* sattvic, rajasic, *and* tamasic. *Find out which category your favorite foods belong to, and how they might be helping or hindering your physical and mental well-being.*

Then you'll read about how different postures and other yoga lifestyle changes can help you with various minor complaints, such as headaches or stomachaches, and even how you can help your body to help itself when you suffer from more serious health conditions, from arthritis to heart disease.

Make yoga a part of your health and vitality.

Chapter 20

Chakras, Mudras, Mantras, and Mandalas

We mention *chakras* many times throughout this book, but in this chapter, we go into more detail about *chakras:* what they are, what they do, and how you can use them to optimize your physical, mental, and spiritual health.

Meet Your *Chakras*

In *yogic* thought, the body contains seven energy centers, called *chakras* (literally "wheels"), that store energy, or the life force, *prana.* Westerners would interpret the *chakras* as nerve centers, but they are much more than this. They are centers of psychospiritual energy that don't precisely correspond to any tangible physical structure.

While the body contains many energy centers and subenergy centers, there are seven primary *chakras* along the midline of the body. Different people have different names for these *chakras* and place them in slightly different locations, but in essence, most agree that these seven *chakras* begin at the base of the spine (where the *kundalini* energy we talked about in Chapter 7, "Can You Breathe?" lies coiled and waiting to be activated) and continue along the spinal cord, ending in the seventh *chakra* at the crown of the head.

Different traditions associate different things with each *chakra:* which body parts, emotions, and thoughts each *chakra* governs; which colors each *chakra* radiates; which areas of our personality each *chakra* represents. We (the authors) like to refer to the *chakras* according to their associated planets, excepting the top two *chakras,* whose names are descriptive.

A Yoga Minute

Every *chakra* has a corresponding color:

Thousand Petaled Lotus	Violet
Sun	Indigo
Mercury	Blue
Venus	Green
Mars	Yellow
Jupiter	Orange
Saturn	Red

Just about everybody who talks about *chakras* calls them something different. There are no pervasive Western names for the *chakras;* people name them after colors, *mantra* syllables, the elements, and so on. Yoga scholar Georg Feuerstein names *chakras* things like "root prop wheel," "jewel city wheel," and "wheel of the unstruck sound." None of these naming systems are arbitrary; the *chakras* do indeed correspond to many different energies. We find the planet-name system to be evocative but nonesoteric—and fun!

Here are the seven *chakras:*

➤ **Saturn *chakra.*** Located just above the anus at the base of the spine, this involves elimination and the sense of smell. This is where the *kundalini* lies. When awakened through yoga, this energy travels up the spine through all the *chakras.*

➤ **Jupiter *chakra.*** Located on the spine near the genitals, this involves water, sexuality, passion, the creation of life, and taste.

➤ **Mars *chakra.*** Located on the spine behind the navel, this is associated with digestion or "gastric fire," your sense of self, and your actions.

➤ **Venus *chakra.*** Located behind the heart, this is the center of your compassion and emotions.

➤ **Mercury *chakra.*** Located in the throat, this is the center for communication.

➤ **Sun *chakra.*** Located in the middle of the brow, this is also known as the *third eye,* or center of unclouded perception.

➤ **Thousand Petaled Lotus *chakra.*** Located at the crown of the skull, this is the center of self-realization, perspective, unity, and enlightenment.

All *chakras* must be activated or awakened for true enlightenment, which is not an easy process. Awakening your *chakras*—releasing the energy that flows through your spine—can take years, perhaps lifetimes! It's hard work to lighten up (or to achieve enlightenment).

The seven chakras *are often depicted as different* mandala-*like shapes drawn along the human spine. More on* mandalas *later in this chapter.*

Ouch!

Feeling frazzled and unfocused? Try a pose that awakens your Saturn *chakra*, located at the base of your spine. Angry, hostile, or overemotional? Try a pose that stimulates your Venus *chakra*, located behind your heart. Having a problem communicating? Work with your Mercury *chakra*, located in the throat. Each *Hatha Yoga* posture is designed to awaken different *chakras*, so practicing the right poses can be the best prescription for what ails you.

Poses to Power Your *Chakras*

Certain yoga poses can make releasing and opening the *chakras* easier. This section talks about a few poses for opening your *chakras*, which floods them with *prana*, energizes them, and helps to balance your entire body/mind. Add a few *chakra*-releasing poses to your yoga routine and feel the power of *prana!*

Prana *Arch*

In this pose, the front of your body opens, releasing tension in your chest, neck, and abdomen. This pose is particularly effective for releasing the *chakras* in the chest and

233

throat. Breathing deeply through this pose encourages the flow of *prana* through the *chakras*.

The prana *arch.*

1. Stand in the mountain pose with your arms hanging loosely at your sides.

2. Inhale as you look up and just slightly behind you. At the same time, lift your hands, palms facing forward, away from your body and out to the sides, as if preparing to give someone a big hug.

3. Contract your buttocks muscles to support your lower back. Don't lean back farther than is comfortable. Breathe deeply several times. Then on an exhale, lower your arms and head, coming back into the mountain pose.

Open Pose

This pose is great for opening the *chakras* in the lower half of the torso. It is also excellent for relaxation and meditation.

The open pose releases the lower chakras.

1. Lie down on the floor on your back with a pillow under your head.

2. Bend your knees and bring the soles of your feet together, letting your knees drop to the floor. If this is uncomfortable, or if the back over-arches, place a pillow under each knee.

3. Bring your palms together in front of your heart, in *namaste*. Breathe deeply several times, focusing on releasing your lower *chakras*. Feel the *prana* flowing through them.

4. If this pose brings strong feelings or emotions to the surface, let them come, feel them, then when you are ready, let them go. Keep breathing and relaxing until you feel calm, energized, and ready to move on.

The Healing Power of *Chakras*

Chakras do more than store energy. Each *chakra* controls a different system of your body as well as a different realm of your emotions. When a *chakra* becomes blocked, you could suffer from health problems—physical or emotional—in that area. For example, a sore throat or an inability to adequately communicate your feelings could signal a blocked Mercury *chakra*. Indigestion or an inability to act on your feelings could mean a blocked Mars *chakra*.

Chakra-at-a-Glance

The following table shows you exactly what each *chakra* controls. Knowing what is linked to what can help you pinpoint the problem, but how do you fix it? Try the earlier *chakra* opening poses, or simply focus on a *chakra* and its associated color during *shavasana* or sitting meditation, to help release, activate, and empower that *chakra*.

Chakra	Color	Location	Physical	Emotional
Saturn	Red	Base of spine	Elimination or releasing, sense of smell	Instinctual responses and drives
Jupiter	Orange	On spine behind the genitals	Reproductive organs, taste, body's water content	Sexuality, passions, creativity
Mars	Yellow	On spine behind the navel	Digestion, taking in or consuming	Actions, sense of self
Venus	Green	On spine behind heart	Cardiovascular system	Compassion, the emotions associated with others
Mercury	Blue	In the throat	Throat, tonsils, voice	Ability to communicate
Sun/ third eye	Indigo (deep blue)	In the middle of the brow	Mental processes, thought, brain	Ability to perceive truth, recognize delusion
Thousand Petaled Lotus	Violet	Crown of your head	Integration of the whole self: body/mind/spirit	Enlightenment

Target Your Chakras *with Yoga Poses*

Depending on which *chakras* are blocked, certain yoga poses throughout this book can help to release and balance those *chakras*. For example, the triangle pose (see the following figure) can help relieve lower back pain by releasing the lower *chakras* and allowing *prana* to flow through this area.

Sometimes the power of two is greater than the power of one. If you have an interested partner, try meditating together, facing each other, legs crossed, knees touching, holding hands. Focus on each of the *chakras* one at a time (perhaps take turns naming each *chakra*, from the Saturn *chakra* all the way up to the Thousand Petaled Lotus *chakra*), or stay silent and meditate individually while connecting physically, emotionally, and energetically through the *chakras* (see the following illustration).

236

The triangle pose.

Connecting your chakras *with a meditation partner.*

Mudra **Magic**

Mudra means "seal," and technically, *mudras* refer to a variety of yoga practices that aren't poses exactly, but techniques for sealing life-force energy inside the body in various ways to preserve it rather than let it escape. These techniques get pretty esoteric and can involve complex rituals, chanting, meditation, and some practices we Westerners might find a little odd.

The word *mudra,* however, is more commonly used today to refer to specific hand gestures used during meditation and *pranayama* to seal the fingers. *Prana* can escape out of the fingertips as it circulates through the body during meditation and *pranayama* exercises, and hand *mudras* bring the fingertips together in various ways for different, subtle effects. Hand *mudras*, in essence, create a *prana* circuit. The energy moves back around and into the body again.

Namaste Mudra: *A Little Respect*

Namaste (pronounced *nah-MAHST*) *mudra,* or the respect gesture, puts the palms together in prayer-like fashion to honor the inner light. Place your palms together and extend your fingers upward, as if you are praying. Hold your hands to your heart. Honor and respect the light within yourself.

Namaste mudra.

Namaste

Om Mudra: *Simply Divine*

Om (pronounced *AUM*) *mudra,* or the divinity gesture, invokes divine balance. Open your palms, and with each hand, bring the tip of your thumb to the tip of your index finger to form a complete circle, which represents the complete cycle and ultimate harmony of divinity. *Om.*

The Om mudra.

OM

Jnana Mudra: *Be a Wise Guy/Gal*

Jnana (pronounced *GAH-nah*) *mudra,* or the wisdom gesture, produces wisdom. Rest your hands, palms up, on your knees, and touch each index finger to the middle of each thumb. The wisdom gesture promotes harmonious inward expression and openness to life's beauty. This *mudra* produces wisdom and encourages the ego to realize that relinquishment brings wisdom. This *mudra* is often practiced during meditation.

The jnana mudra.

Buddhi Mudra: *How Enlightening!*

Buddhi mudra, or enlightenment gesture, is often associated with the Buddha, and is ideal for centering and calming. Bring your thumb and index finger together, tip to tip, as in the *Om mudra.* Then bring both hands together, knuckles touching, and rest your hands against your lower abdomen at your Jupiter *chakra.* This *mudra* represents divinity and the oneness of self and also the joining of all energies. It quiets the mind, stills action, and enlightens the self to its inner divinity. Try this *mudra* when you are feeling tense or rushed.

The buddhi mudra.

Mantras: **Beyond** *Om*

"I'll do yoga," you say, "but I draw the line at chanting." Okay, so you've been put off by a few *Om* stereotypes on television and in movies. But bear with us for just a little bit—it's not as bad as you think, once you understand what chanting is all about.

A *mantra* is a sound or sounds that resonate in the body and evoke certain energies. *Mantras* help stimulate the *chakras* by soothing your mind and awakening your senses.

Om is a common *mantra* because it's designed to invoke a universal perspective: You see your body/mind in relation to its place in the big picture. In Sanskrit, *Om* is spelled "aum," and each letter is a sacred symbol:

> ➤ **a** represents the self in the material world.

> ➤ **u** represents the psychic realm.

> ➤ **m** represents indwelling spiritual light.

Chanting *Om* unifies your perceptions so you can sense yourself as an integral part of the universe.

Wise Yogi Tells Us

Om Shanti Shanti Shanti (pronounced *OHM SHAHN-tee SHAHN-tee SHAHN-tee*) is a great beginning *mantra* to try. *Shanti* means "peace," and when repeated three times, it balances the body, mind, and spirit. It's easy to use and to remember.

Gradually, the chant helps you shed everything that separates you from the universe —all your negativity, illusions, and misperceptions of yourself and the world. *Om* is a great *mantra* for anyone. Don't be embarrassed! Give it a try!

Know Your Sanskrit

A **mantra** is a sacred sound used in meditation as the object of focus, meant to resonate within the body and awaken the *chakras.* The word *mantra* is a composite of two Sanskrit root words. The first word, *man,* means "continual or constant thinking." The second word, *tra,* means "to be free." *Mantra* is a process by which you free yourself from worries or doubts, but not from consciousness.

But as we said, *Om* isn't the only *mantra.* Many Sanskrit word combinations serve as common *mantras,* but any sequence of words meaningful to you can be a *mantra.* You might find something that works for you in the following list:

➤ Light (inhalation), love (exhalation). Love (inhalation), light (exhalation).

➤ One is all, all is one.

➤ *Om namah sivaya* (pronounced *OHM NAH-mah SHE-vah-yah*). (Note: *Siva* destroys and recreates. The energy that destroys the lower self builds the higher self.)

➤ Amen.

➤ Hallelujah.

➤ *Om Shanti Shanti Shanti* (pronounced *OHM SHAHN-tee,* meaning all peace, peace, peace).

➤ *Hari Om* (pronounced *HA-ree OHM,* meaning removing fear, uncovering bliss).

➤ *Hong Sau* (pronounced *HONG SAW,* meaning the holy breath; inhale *"hong,"* exhale *"sau"*).

Mandalas: Goin' 'Round in Circles

While a *mantra* is meant to soothe the body and mind through sound, a *mandala* is meant to center the mind through sight. *Mandalas* are beautiful, usually circular, geometric designs that draw your eye to the center. *Mandala* means "circle" or "center," and the designs suggest the circular patterns that exist in so many levels of life, from atoms to solar systems. *Mandalas* represent a pilgrimage to enlightenment. As you focus on the center of the *mandala,* you'll notice the outer parts shifting and changing in your peripheral vision; eventually, your focus will become clear, and the center will be all that you see.

Know Your Sanskrit

A **mandala** is a circular geometric design used as a center of focus in meditation and meant to suggest the universe's circular motif (from atoms to solar systems) and the spirit's journey. *Mandala* means "circle" or "center."

Mandalas *are a metaphor for the spiritual path of the mind and body. This well-known man-*dala *is built into the floor of Chartres Cathedral in France. Spiritual pilgrims literally walked through the* mandala *to attain spiritual insight. Get a pencil and try walking the Chartres* mandala *by tracing the path you would take to reach the center and then return from the center to the world again.*

Using *mandalas* and *mantras* together is a wonderful way to meditate, because the combination of aural and visual stimulation awakens and clarifies your mind, body, and spirit in multiple ways. Adding color to your *mandala* goes even further toward stimulating the senses. (And you thought meditation would be boring!)

The Least You Need to Know

➤ *Chakras* are energy centers in your body that govern different areas of your physical, emotional, and spiritual self.

➤ Unblocking and releasing *chakras* through meditation and targeted yoga poses can improve your physical, emotional, and spiritual health.

➤ *Mantras* are words or groups of words meant to resonate within the body for certain effects and are often used as an aural focus in meditation. The most well-known *mantra* is the Sanskrit word *Om*.

➤ *Mandalas* are circular patterns meant to focus the vision and, by extension, the consciousness during meditation. Combining *mantras* and *mandalas* in meditation results in an even more powerful centering effect.

Chapter 21

You Are What You Eat

In This Chapter

➤ Three types of foods bring out three types of personal qualities

➤ Moderate eating is best

➤ The benefits of a lacto vegetarian diet

Now that you've got a handle on yoga's basic principles and are happily posturing away, let's consider another extremely important but often overlooked aspect of yoga: diet. It only makes sense that if your body, mind, and spirit are one, how you feed your body will influence the whole package. Western scientists have long recognized that a healthy diet is crucial to good health, although through the decades the definition of "healthy" has certainly changed.

Gunas Gracious!

A fundamental principle is the yoga diet's primary influence. *Yogis* have traditionally divided food (and everything else, but we'll just talk about food in this chapter) into three categories, called *gunas*. The three *gunas* are *sattva, rajas,* and *tamas,* and each represents a different type of energy. When applied to food, these energies go into our bodies and affect us in different ways, making us more balanced, or imbalanced, depending on our individual needs and the food we eat. *Sattvic* food promotes health, vitality, strength, and tranquillity; *rajasic* food promotes excessive energy, agitation, and discontentment; and *tamasic* food promotes lethargy, laziness, and inactivity.

Imagine a teeter-totter. The three *gunas* exist along the board of the teeter-totter, with *rajas* on one end, *tamas* on the other end, and *sattva* squarely in the middle. For example, if you tend to be a *rajasic* type of person, or you eat a lot of *rajasic* food (such as meat, hot peppers, double espressos, and other stimulating kinds of foods), and then you eat *tamasic* food (such as processed or preserved food or alcohol), you could achieve an uneasy balance, like two kids standing on either side of the teeter-totter. The slightest shift, and both kids will topple.

But what if the two kids sit right over the teeter-totter's fulcrum? They'll be pretty stable, and that is what *sattvic* food—such as fresh, organic fruits, vegetables, and grains in or close to their natural state (and other *sattvic* influences like a regular schedule, plenty of sleep, and a steady routine)—does for your body. It balances you in a stable way. Your health will be much less likely to topple. You'll find the state of *samyama* much more accessible.

Achieve a sattvic *balance for good yoga nutrition.*

TAMAS   SATTVA   RAJAS

Samyama is what *yogis* strive for. It means holding your consciousness together through concentration, meditation, and contemplation in an attempt to understand everything about the object of your investigation, whether that is poetry, the study of medicine, or the study of yoga postures. *Samyama* is the final state that results from the active process of learning. In other words, it is total absorption in your activity, and in your life itself.

On the other hand, *duhkha* is what often leads us astray. *Duhkha* is a feeling of discomfort or pain, suffering, sickness, or simply mental limitation. It is that deep-down feeling that something is wrong or out of place. *Duhkha* keeps you from achieving *samyama*. It makes you feel like you don't have the ability or are somehow inadequate—not healthy enough or strong enough or smart enough. *Duhkha* can arise out of excessive desire for something—even for enlightenment! It can be likened to a mental "virus" that infects your attitude and progress. *Duhkha* is like balancing on the end of the teeter-totter. You may be level at the moment, but it doesn't feel very good or secure. You are in fear of falling.

Know Your Sanskrit

Samyama (pronounced *SAHM–YAH–mah*) is a state that exists when concentration, meditation, and contemplation are all producing a perfectly balanced, concentrated meditational state. *Sam* means "together," and *yama* means "discipline." **Duhkha** (*DOO-kah*) is pain, suffering, trouble, and discomfort. From *dur*, which means "bad," and *kha*, which means "axle hole" or "space" (hence, being in a bad space), *duhkha* is a mental state during which limitations and a profound sense of "wrongness" are perceived. *Duhkha* holds us back from self–actualization.

So how are *samyama* and *duhkha* related to the three *gunas?* Too many *rajasic* and/or *tamasic* foods produce *duhkha*, that's how! Balance is maintained with *sattvic* foods, and in fact, yoga itself can be seen as a process of "sattvification." It helps keep you *duhkha*-free.

So we know we want to maintain a *sattvic* state of mind as often as possible. What better way than to eat a *sattvic* diet? Since feeding the body is akin to feeding the mind, *sattvic* food will encourage a *sattvic* mental state once we are balanced. However, *sattvic* foods won't necessarily be able to balance someone who is naturally very *rajasic* or *tamasic*. For instance, a very *tamasic* person, one who has very little energy and leads a sedentary life, may find that a little *rajasic* food like coffee or a nice hot salsa can help restore a balance. Then *sattvic* food makes a great "maintenance diet." A swinging pendulum isn't easy to stop. The way it best comes to rest is by a slow change in the intensity of its swing.

What's Your Nature?

As we mentioned, the *gunas* don't just apply to food. They are qualities that can be applied to the universe in general. The mind is made up of these three states. *Tamas* is dullness, lassitude, and constancy. *Rajas* is activity and agitation. *Sattva* is clarity, tranquillity, and compassion. These three states also represent the three states of personal evolution: first the mind is dull, then it becomes active, and then, ideally, it finds true compassion.

The wild activity of *rajas* is considered on a higher plane than the inert *tamas*, because without activity, one cannot reach compassion (*sattva*). Most people swing around from quality to quality, experiencing each at different points in their lives, even throughout the day. However, one aspect is usually dominant in each person's personality.

Yes, one of these qualities is probably dominant in you. Knowing which is your type can help you to balance yourself. If you're a typical *rajas*-natured Westerner, for example, you can consciously minimize or eliminate *rajasic* food from your diet, replacing it with *sattvic* food. You'll probably notice a distinct difference in the way you feel—calmer, clearer, and less agitated.

Not sure which type you are? Take this mini-quiz to get a better picture of yourself:

1. If I'm feeling under a lot of stress, I'll be most likely to …

   a. Go take a nap. At least I'll be able to forget about it all for a while.

   b. Pace back and forth, worrying and wasting time.

   c. Analyze why I'm under stress and make a plan to deal with it.

2. I would describe my diet as …

   a. Centered around my food addictions: caffeine, sugar, or salt. Meals are really important to me because I have to have my food! It would be very difficult for me to give up any food I love.

   b. Very irregular. I grab a bite of whatever is handiest when I have the time. Sometimes I forget to eat or am so stressed out that I eat way too much without realizing it.

   c. Healthy, well-balanced, with lots of fruits and vegetables. Not a big fan of meat.

3. In my personal relationships, I tend to be …

   a. The passive one.

   b. The dominant one.

   c. Fairly equal with the others in my life.

If you answered mostly As, you're probably *tamas*-natured. You'd rather lie on the couch than go for a jog; you tend to get addicted to pleasurable things like sugar, cigarettes, or coffee; and you have a hard time getting things done. You may have difficulty getting yourself into a habit of practicing yoga postures, but yoga will be of great benefit to you, revving up your system, increasing your energy level, and giving you the get-up-and-go you need to get through the day.

If you answered mostly Bs, you're probably *rajas*-natured. You're typically overwrought, excited, anxious, or agitated. You get a lot done and fast, but you have a hard time relaxing and quieting your mind. For you, meditation is a real challenge, but you could really use the skill of being able to calm that overactive mind of yours. If you suffer from insomnia, regular yoga practice can help you sleep. In fact, regular practice of anything is good for the impetuous and routine-resistant *rajas*-natured.

If you answered mostly Cs, you tend to be *sattvic*-natured. You adhere to the sensible notion of moderation in many aspects of your life, and the *yogic* lifestyle will probably be relatively easy for you to adopt. You find a sense of peace in yoga postures, you find meditation enjoyable, and you already follow the *yogic* diet without even intending to! In fact, you may wonder why you haven't discovered yoga before now.

Wise Yogi Tells Us

Feeling stressed out? Gently heat one cup of low-fat milk on the stove or in the microwave. Pour it into a mug and add one tablespoon of honey and a pinch of dried ginger. Stir, find a comfy seat, and relax. Sip slowly. Ahhhhh! Don't drink milk? Cut a two-inch slice of fresh gingerroot, peel it, and slice it into disks. Put it in the bottom of a mug or cup, and pour boiling water over it. Let it steep for about five minutes, then remove the ginger. Add a squeeze of fresh lemon juice and a tablespoon of honey. Mmmm!

Yogi *Food*

So let's cut to the chase: What kind of food is *sattvic* food? *Sattvic* foods are pure foods. Most foods that are fresh, organically grown, additive- and preservative-free, unprocessed, and alkaline are considered *sattvic*. These include the following:

➤ Fresh fruits and juices

➤ Most fresh vegetables

➤ Whole-grain cereals

➤ Nuts and seeds, especially almonds and sesame seeds

➤ Pulses (dried peas, beans, and lentils)

➤ Milk and milk products (unfermented), including butter

➤ Honey

A Yoga Minute

Traditionally, milk has been an important part of the *yogi*'s diet and has always been considered *sattvic*. However, milk today is not what it used to be. Factory farms with their hormone- and antibiotic-laden cows packed in tiny stalls in sunless enclosures, pasteurization, and shipment to supermarkets in plastic packaging have all compromised milk's *sattvic* nature. In addition, many people are lactose intolerant, meaning that they lack the enzyme necessary for the body to digest milk.

Sattvic foods help you think more clearly, because your body is unclouded and unhindered by impurities, chemicals, and stimulants. *Sattvic* foods promote contemplative thought, vitality, energy, tranquillity, happiness, and overall health. Most serious yoga practitioners exist primarily on *sattvic* foods, although because food in and of itself is not an obsession for the healthy *yogi,* occasional tastes of other foods when these are offered aren't a problem. The wise *yogi* eats moderately, and moderation means *not* being obsessive about anything, even moderation!

If you're unable to drink milk or choose to avoid all dairy products (a truly nonviolent approach to eating), simply update our list of *sattvic* foods by eliminating milk. Stick with organic produce and whole grains, the foods that remain *sattvic* even in our complicated world.

Wise Yogi Tells Us

If you aren't ready for all-out vegetarianism, try it for a day. Tell yourself you can have a cheeseburger tomorrow, but today you'll stick with hearty split-pea soup over rice or a steaming plate of pasta with sautéed mushrooms. Tomorrow, before your cheeseburger, notice how you feel. Lighter? Hungrier? No different? Calmer? Then try it again next week.

Pungent, Spicy Westerners

As we've mentioned, most Westerners tend to be *rajas*-natured because Western life is so *rajas*-oriented. Our culture rewards high energy, overachievement, even anxiety and agitation if they help to get the job done! *Rajasic* foods are generally the stimulating kind: spicy, sour, pungent, and bitter. The following are examples of *rajasic* food:

➤ All meat

➤ All fish

➤ Eggs

➤ Hot peppers

➤ Most strong spices, especially black and red pepper

➤ Coffee, tea, cola, and other stimulating, caffeine-laden beverages

Ancient cultures often fed their warriors meat before sending them off to battle, because it was known that meat increased aggression and agitation. After a good meat-fest, warriors could fight and kill better. Assuming you don't have the need to fight and kill anyone, however, why not try cutting down or even eliminating most *rajasic* foods from your diet? You may find a new sense of calm and a clearer head.

Of course, a little *rajasic* food now and then won't hurt anyone. It's what you do most of the time that counts. But if you exist on steak and eggs, or spicy beef burritos, or sausage-and-pepper sandwiches, or coffee and diet cola, even a non*yogi* can tell you that you aren't going to be at your healthiest.

Stale Leftovers for Couch Potatoes

Tamasic food is considered impure and includes anything stale, old, aged, fermented, spoiled, overly processed, preservative-filled, or addictive. Here are some examples of *tamasic* food:

➤ Coffee, tea, cola, and other sources of caffeine (on this list, too, because they are both stimulating and addictive).

➤ Alcohol, including wine and beer.

➤ Aged cheese, yogurt, other fermented dairy products.

➤ Foods that are canned, pickled, highly salted.

➤ Tobacco (we know, you smoke it, you don't eat it—but it still counts!).

➤ Any food that's been sitting around too long, even if it still looks good (for example, produce that has been heavily sprayed and waxed so it can last through a journey across country and long periods of storage).

➤ Anything processed, packaged, frozen, or preserved, from that "lite" microwavable dinner to that box of snack cakes that would last in your pantry for five years.

Tamasic foods dull your mind. They make you feel tired and sap your ambition and strength (just what the preserving process—*tamasa*-fying!—does to fresh, or *sattvic,* food). Too much *tamasic* food will drain away your energy and your vitality, eventually bringing on a lack of joy in life, if not serious illness. No matter how much coloring and how many preservatives are added to make the food look good, when our bodies ingest it, the "makeup" comes right off and the food's true quality is revealed.

A Yoga Minute

Maybe you're wondering how caffeine can be both *rajasic* and *tamasic*. The stimulating quality of caffeine—that "buzz" that shifts you into high gear—is, indeed, *rajasic*, but there's more to caffeine than its stimulating nature. Coffee, tea, and cola are also addictive, and addictive substances are *tamasic*. The habitual nature of caffeine woos the *tamas*-natured; plus, the stimulating effect gets hard-to-move *tamas*-natured folks up on their feet and out the door to work. Yes, yes, we understand. You *love* your cup of coffee! (We love ours, too.) Fear not. Remember, it's what you do most of the time that counts. If the rest of your diet is basically *sattvic*, an occasional cup of coffee isn't going to hurt.

Unfortunately, many Westerners are addicted to *tamasic* food, especially sources of caffeine and alcohol. Also, we've been tricked into believing we don't have time for anything but preservative-laden "convenience" food. Our supermarkets are brimming with *tamasic* fare, but that doesn't mean you have to put it in your grocery cart. A stock of tomato soup or commercial spaghetti sauce will keep longer than a stock of fresh tomatoes, but it certainly isn't better, or worth the price!

Moderation in All Things (As If You Didn't Know!)

But wait! Just because you now know which foods are best for you doesn't mean you should throw down this book, run to the kitchen, and start indulging. Calm down, you *rajas*-natured ones. Don't plan your indulgent feast just yet, you *tamas*-natured folk. Cultivating *sattva* means more than shoveling in massive quantities of the "right" foods. It also involves a few principles of eating:

➤ **Eat slowly.** Chew each bite 50 times (or, if that's just too much to ask, start with 10 times and work your way up). Taste your food. Don't think about what you're going to eat next or what you need to do next. Give your meal some time. Give each bite some time.

➤ **Eat with full attention to eating.** That means no TV, no newspaper, and no trance-like gazing at the back of the cereal box, fascinating as it may be.

➤ **Enjoy your food and savor the eating experience.** Live in the moment of your meal!

➤ **Don't eat too much.** Try to leave the table with a little room left in your stomach.

➤ **Don't eat too often.** That means avoiding between-meal snacking, late-night binges, and 3:00 A.M. Dagwood sandwiches.

If food is too important to you, it will control you. If you have a food addiction, you already know what it's like to be controlled. Food is meant to keep you alive and to enhance your existence; food isn't meant to fill emotional voids.

Overindulgence taxes your body, and it's been suggested that regular and consistent undereating (not undernourishment—an important distinction) increases longevity. That means more time on this earth for practicing yoga, and more time to enjoy the improved you. Remember the old and familiar adage (did your parents ever tell you this?), "Moderation in All Things." This is a seriously important concept. Live moderately and you'll live well.

Wise Yogi Tells Us

If you have habitual *tamasic* tendencies (to food, cigarettes, caffeine, or whatever), we recommend *The Complete Idiot's Guide to Breaking Bad Habits, Second Edition,* by Suzanne LeVert and Gary McClain, Ph.D. (Alpha Books, 2001). Check it out!

Sometimes the best way to let food work for you is to give your body a rest from food. Moderate eating is great, but sometimes even the moderate eater can benefit from a short juice fast. Occasional one-day juice fasts (nothing but fresh fruit and vegetable juice) are excellent system cleansers. However, fasting should not be overdone. Remember, moderation!

Another great and easy way to fast is to eat a healthy breakfast, a hearty lunch, and an early, light supper, then not to eat anything but juice and water after 5:00 P.M. (Some people prefer to fast after 3:00 P.M.—an effective weight-loss and system-cleansing tool if you don't mind skipping dinner.)

If you fast too often or for too long, or fast while only drinking water, you're committing violence on your own body (and that isn't following the *yama* of *ahimsa,* or nonviolence!). Before altering your diet or performing a fast, consult your physician or a licensed dietitian to come up with the best nutritional plan for your individual health and fitness needs.

If you do suffer from food addictions, breaking them can be extremely difficult. Maybe you can't even imagine shelving your life-sustaining coffee mug. Maybe you binge on cookies every weekend or are seemingly incapable of passing a fast-food restaurant without driving through for a double cheeseburger and fries.

Ouch!

If you are fasting and experience headaches, dizziness, or other discomfort beyond mild hunger, give yourself a break, practice nonviolence, and have something to eat. Fasting is not about hurting yourself. When breaking a fast, make sure you begin eating gradually again. Start with soup, bread, a salad, or something else natural (close to its natural state) and light in fat and calories.

We have a nice little secret for you: You don't have to feel guilty. You don't have to deprive yourself (just yet!). All you have to do is practice all the *other* aspects of yoga: the postures, the breathing, the meditation. Here's where yoga works its magic. Yoga is transformative. It changes you. If you diligently practice it, within a few weeks or months, you'll be able to enjoy a cup of coffee without needing more or feeling addicted. Or maybe you won't want it at all. You won't feel the need for the caffeine. Fresh fruit will seem far more luscious than a bag of processed, store-bought cookies. And fast food will seem downright ... barbaric?

The point is, you don't really need to try to change your habits. You don't need to suffer and strive. If you're disciplined in the other areas of yoga, yoga will help you with the rest.

C'mon, Vegetarian?

Okay, we'll say it again: Here's where yoga works its magic. Yoga is transformative. It changes you.

Westerners are funny about vegetarianism. They seem to fall into two camps. There's the "Of *course* I'm a vegetarian. Aren't *you?*" camp, and the "You aren't *actually* one of those *vegetarians,* are you?" camp. Even if you're a vegetarian and don't judge meat-eaters, or a meat-eater who doesn't judge vegetarians, many who don't share your views about meat will assume you're in the "opposite camp" and will be on the defensive.

We aren't sure why this antagonistic scenario has developed in the West, but it has. If you're a vegetarian or have tried without success to quit eating meat, you have surely encountered "the attitude." Also, if you eat meat but know a lot of vegetarians, you may have felt similarly maligned.

So let's all try, just for a minute, to let go of all that. Let's be objective, as far as that's possible. Do you like meat? Could you do without it? Aside from what anyone else in the world might think, does the idea of a vegetarian diet appeal to you? Although some *yogis* are *vegans* and some are *fruitarians,* the most common *yogi* diet is a *lacto vegetarian* diet. What exactly *is* a vegetarian, then, you ask? *Vegetarian* is a blanket term, and there are indeed several *kinds* of vegetarians. Check out this vegetarian primer, and you'll be an expert on the variety and range of vegetarian diets!

➤ **Lacto vegetarians** don't eat any meat, poultry, fish, or eggs. Their diets consist primarily of fruits, vegetables, whole grains (like rice, oats, and wheat), pasta, nuts, seeds, pulses (dried beans, peas, and lentils), milk, and milk products.

➤ **Lacto ovo vegetarians** are the same as lacto vegetarians but also eat eggs.

➤ **Vegans** eat no animal substance of any kind, including all dairy products. Diligent vegans even avoid eating things like gelatin and other products made with preservatives or other ingredients made from animal parts (like rennet), and wearing leather or other clothing made from animals.

➤ **Fruitarians** eat primarily fruit, but also some vegetables. The primary rule for fruitarians is that all food must be consumed raw. Yes, that means avoiding *all* cooked foods!

There are a lot of great reasons to practice a vegetarian diet:

➤ A vegetarian diet is in harmony with *ahimsa,* the *niyama* of nonviolence.

➤ A vegetarian diet is healthier for your heart, because it tends to be low in cholesterol and saturated fat.

➤ According to many wise *yogis,* when an animal is slaughtered, it is filled with intense fear and anxiety. Eating that meat transfers the terrible fear to you.

➤ A vegetarian diet makes many people feel lighter, more energetic, and healthier. Physical activity becomes less of an effort, and food becomes less of an obsession.

But what if your answer to the question of whether you could eat from the lacto vegetarian menu is a resounding "No way!"? As we said before, don't force yourself to do anything you aren't yet ready to do. You can certainly be committed to yoga without being committed to vegetarianism. In fact, many yoga teachers don't encourage vegetarianism or any dietary modification, especially to their Western students. These teachers know that yoga will do that job on its own, when the time is right.

Many *yogis* start out without any intention of becoming vegetarians, but the more yoga transforms them, the less interested they are in meat, until finally, one day … poof! … another vegetarian is born. Simply deciding to become a vegetarian will not magically grant you a kind heart. Plenty of mean-spirited vegetarians are walking around out there in the world! Vegetarianism doesn't make you a *yogi;* yoga leads you to nonviolence, which may eventually lead you to vegetarianism. Maybe this day is in your near future, and maybe it's a long, long way off. It's your journey. What's right for you is unique, and only you can truly

Wise Yogi Tells Us

Some meat-eaters feel guilty eating meat in front of vegetarians, and some vegetarians feel guilty because they don't want their meat-eating friends to feel guilty. The true *yogic* way is not to judge others or yourself harshly. Yoga is a path of loving acceptance. No guilt, no condescension. Pure joy.

determine your own course. So consider vegetarianism, be open to the idea, but if it just isn't "you" (or at least, the "you" you are today), let it go. Maybe it will come back to surprise you when you're ready for it.

Vegetarian or not, do try to eat a healthy, fresh, primarily *sattvic* diet. Everyone can agree that fresh, whole, unprocessed food is a delight to eat. A diet of *sattvic* food makes living so much nicer, yoga practice so much easier, and may even make this wonderful life of yours a little bit longer and a little bit more wonderful.

The Least You Need to Know

➤ Different types of foods—*sattvic, rajasic,* and *tamasic*—have different effects on you.

➤ Fresh, whole, unprocessed food helps you think more clearly. Stimulating food can agitate you, and stale or preservative-filled food can sap your energy.

➤ Moderation in all things is best!

➤ A lacto vegetarian diet has many health-related and spiritual benefits.

Chapter 22

Rx: Yoga

> ### In This Chapter
>
> ➤ Your body has many layers, or levels, of existence
>
> ➤ How yoga can help your nagging complaints
>
> ➤ How yoga can help when your condition is more serious

If you're human (which we assume you all are), chances are you've experienced illness and pain in your lifetime. Even if you've never been seriously ill, you've certainly had a cold, the flu, maybe insomnia, possibly indigestion, an occasional headache, an aching back. Our human bodies are far from perfectly functioning, especially considering how much and how vigorously we use them. But pain and discomfort aren't necessarily par for the course in the life of a *yogi*. The *yogi* has a few tricks, and you, as a novice *yogi*, are privy to this health-inspiring information. Read on for how to help prevent, relieve, and sometimes even cure your health problems.

What Makes You Sick?

Theories abound concerning the cause of illness and pain, but many *yogis* believe that although illness can be caused by physical factors such as viruses, bacteria, and accidents, illness can also be brought on or encouraged by ...

> ➤ Insufficient *prana,* or life force, within the body.
>
> ➤ Too much *rajasic* (causing agitation) and/or *tamasic* (causing lethargy) food.
>
> ➤ Lack of cleanliness.
>
> ➤ Unhappiness.
>
> ➤ Pessimism and negativity.

➤ An imbalance within the physical body or the mind, which can be caused by any of these factors.

One of the characteristics of conventional, or *allopathic,* medicine is that it tends to pinpoint and isolate a problem or symptom and treat it, and it alone, which is sometimes just what the body needs. The body is like a machine that occasionally requires the repair of a specific part (a broken bone, a clogged heart, a ruptured appendix).

Know Your Sanskrit

Svasthya (pronounced SVAH-sthyah) is the Sanskrit word for health, from *sva-stha,* which means "one's own state." **Roga** (ROH-gah) means "sickness," and **vyadhi** (VYAH-dee) means "disease."

Holistic medicine tends to first look at the "big picture," or the whole person. What are you doing that could be causing your illness (*roga*), pain, or disease (*vyadhi*)? Who are you? How is your general health (*svasthya*)? What is your health history? How is your posture? What is your attitude? What is your view of life? Holistic medicine seeks the answers to all these questions in an effort to find the source of a problem, rather than merely treating the symptoms of a condition or illness.

Yoga, too, takes this holistic approach to your health. Yoga treatments are great when used in conjunction with traditional healthcare, because such an approach results in an all-encompassing treatment. Yoga works on your body and your mind to free them of impurities and imbalances that could cause health problems for you later.

Body Beyond the Body: The Five Sheaths of Existence

In Chapter 8, "*Hatha Yoga:* May the Force Be with You," we briefly mentioned the five sheaths of existence, but they're worth touching on again here because they're intimately connected with the state of your health. The first sheath consists of your physical body. The second is the vital body, made of *prana,* the life force. The third sheath is your mind, including your emotions and thoughts. The fourth sheath is your higher intellect, and the fifth sheath is the bliss sheath, filled with positive energy and inner peace. Being human means we originally existed in the bliss sheath, and we have to work our way down into the physical body, then find our way back out to the bliss sheath again.

Disturbances or imbalances in any of your body's sheaths, not just the physical layer, can result in illness. Neglecting your nutritional needs, for example, could cause an imbalance in your physical body, which could, in turn, result in an imbalance of *prana,* which could make you feel uncomfortable and stressed. When you don't feel well, maybe you begin to think more negatively, causing an imbalance in your third sheath of existence. Pretty soon, you're all out of whack!

Disturbances of the third, or mind, sheath can also arise when strong feelings distort your inner balance. Maybe you're fixated on your dislike of a colleague at work. You spend a lot of time fuming about what he said or what she did. Pretty soon, you aren't breathing productively, and your second sheath becomes disturbed. Then you get a cold, and your first sheath is unbalanced.

Even positive behavior can cause an imbalance when taken to an extreme. Perhaps you absolutely love running—normally a healthy activity—so much that you spend all your time running at the expense of all other activities and interests. Your mind becomes obsessed with running and loses interest in other aspects of life. You lose friends because everyone is tired of hearing about running. Your body begins to suffer because you lose too much weight or injure your legs or feet. See how it's all connected?

Even the practice of yoga *asanas* can become an obsession. If you spend all your time on yoga poses and neglect the other areas of your life, you'll throw yourself out of balance.

The "moderation in all things" adage comes into play in health as well as in diet. Anything you do to an extreme will cause an imbalance in your body and mind, or in your first three sheaths of existence. Remember *ahimsa*, or nonviolence? Practice it by refusing to commit violence to your body with obsessive actions. Also, observe *santosha*, or contentment, by practicing satisfaction, peace, and tranquillity. You'll have a much easier time staying obsession-free.

Yoga for Those Nagging Complaints

When your physical complaints are relatively minor but persistent, yoga can be great therapy. You'll probably find that with regular, consistent yoga practice, you'll suffer less often from minor complaints. If they do arise, however, try a few appropriate yoga *asanas* (postures) and stick with your yoga rules for living (*yamas* and *niyamas*) for effective relief.

Oh, My Aching Back ...

Because we all walk around upright, our backs are bound to suffer. Our poor spines carry all that weight around and are continually jarred by the pounding of our feet, not to mention twisted and contorted by less-than-perfect posture. Weak stomach muscles are a common cause of back pain. Injury to a disk or vertebrae can cause back pain. Yoga can help in these cases. If you suffer from back pain, include the following exercises, which strengthen the stomach and/or tone the spine, in your yoga routine:

➤ Cobra pose (Chapter 14, "Bending Over Backbends")

➤ Single leg lifts (Chapter 16, "A Continuous Flow")

➤ Boat pose (Chapter 18, "Take the Forward Path")

A Yoga Minute

Back-pain sufferers may need more calcium and magnesium. Great sources are milk, yo-gurt, cheese, dark leafy greens like collard greens and kale, calcium-fortified orange juice, almonds, calcium-fortified tofu, broccoli, wheat bran, wheat germ, whole-wheat flour, calcium-fortified cereal, dried beans, peanut butter, and dried apricots. If you have a spine-related injury, however, be sure to check with your doctor before trying any yoga postures. Once your doctor gives the go-ahead, practice under the supervision of an experienced teacher to be sure you perform the poses correctly and don't injure yourself further.

Oh, My Aching Head ...

It's the rare individual indeed who can say he or she has never suffered from a head-ache. Unfortunately, it's often difficult to find the source of a headache. Headaches can be caused by a negative reaction to a certain food, air pollution, allergies, sinus problems, eyestrain, stress, and any number of other factors. Try eliminating sus-pected sources of regular headaches, such as caffeine, poor posture, or a particular food. If your headache is severe or your headache patterns change, see a doctor. For occasional, irregular headaches, however, your best bet may be to step up your yoga practice to put your body in the best possible condition for curing itself.

For headache relief, try the following:

➤ Try the breathing techniques in Chapter 7, "Can You Breathe?"

➤ Gently rotate and flex your neck and toes.

➤ Practice inverted postures where your head is lowered briefly. These may help a headache, because inverted postures increase the flow of oxygen to the brain.

➤ Make sure you maintain a balanced diet. Decrease or eliminate your intake of nuts, aged cheeses, chocolate, caffeine, and food containing nitrates (like lunch-eon meats and hot dogs). These foods produce allergy-like reactions in many people.

Why Am I So Tired?

Fatigue is a common problem in our overextended and fast-paced lives. Sometimes we simply wear ourselves out! Fatigue can also be caused by stress and extreme mental exertion, such as when you've been studying excessively, or when you're bothered by an emotional problem, such as depression or anxiety. A good holistic healthcare practitioner or therapist may be able to help you discover the underlying cause of your fatigue. If you notice unusual fatigue, however, even when you've gotten enough sleep, consult a physician.

For occasional bouts of fatigue during the day, a 20-minute power nap can work wonders. If you aren't in a position to take a nap, try …

➤ Practicing *shavasana,* or the corpse pose, for five minutes (see Chapter 19, "Dead to the World").

➤ Doing deep-breathing exercises to replenish your *prana.*

➤ Any of the backbends in Chapter 14 to help energize you.

Wise Yogi Tells Us

A few lifestyle modifications could be the answer to eliminating fatigue in your life. Try …

➤ Getting off caffeine ASAP!

➤ Not eating anything sweet before noon.

➤ Eating a low-fat diet. Too much fat slows you down and wears you out.

➤ Maintaining a positive attitude. Don't sweat the small stuff!

Why Can't I Sleep?

On the other hand, we have the insomniacs. If you have trouble getting to sleep, common sense will probably tell you to lay off the caffeine, especially in the evening, and not to eat a whole pepperoni pizza at midnight. Stress is a common cause of insomnia, too. How can you sleep if your mind is abuzz with the worries of the day? Maybe you aren't purposefully sabotaging your body's ability to snooze, but if you nevertheless can't seem to catch even a few winks, try the following:

➤ Meditate. Evening meditation can calm and still your mind, making sleep easier. Many wise *yogis* sit in full lotus in meditation so that if—or when—they fall asleep, they won't fall over!

➤ *Shavasana* is as good for insomnia as it is for fatigue. See Chapter 19.

➤ Forward bends quiet the body and mind. Try any of the poses from Chapter 18.

➤ To help you get to sleep, take a warm bath before bed, and don't eat for at least six hours before bedtime.

➤ Dried lavender in your bath or stuffed in your pillowcase can help soothe you to sleep.

What's Up with My Digestion?

The digestive system is tricky. Maybe you've noticed you can eat chili dogs, cotton candy, and ice cream all day some days and feel fine, while on other days, a few bites of an enchilada are all it takes to give you heartburn all night long. Part of the reason is that much of your digestive success depends on the manner in which you eat. If you eat slowly, concentrate on your food, and enjoy the experience, you'll have a better chance at digesting without a hitch. Rushed, stressed eating or eating when you aren't hungry or aren't feeling well will lead you down a short path to indigestion.

Some people have chronic digestive problems, which could signal a number of possible health issues. If you suffer from frequent heartburn, indigestion, bloating, gas, or stomach cramps after eating, see your doctor. Occasional cases can be alleviated by a few good yoga poses.

➤ Try *shavasana*. (See Chapter 19.)

➤ Poses that move the digestive area through compression and opening are good for improving digestion. Try the fish pose (Chapter 14), which lengthens the abdomen, followed by the child's pose (Chapter 18), which compresses the abdomen.

➤ The Sun Salutation (Chapter 16) is an excellent flowing series of poses to move and open the digestive system.

Wise Yogi Tells Us

If you don't seem to have a particular problem other than the simple presence of lots of stress, practice deep breathing to increase the production of endorphins in your system. Endorphins are the body's natural painkillers and will help lower your blood pressure and heart rate.

This Cold Won't Go Away ...

Having a cold all winter long is frustrating as well as counterproductive to your happiness and well-being. If you can't get rid of your cold or keep getting colds back-to-back, consider where the virus is coming from. Are you washing your hands often enough? Do you frequently touch your face? Are you in contact with a lot of people all day long?

During the cold season, cold germs are everywhere, so be extra careful about hygiene. If you have kids, make sure they wash their hands before they eat and before they touch food others will eat. Remind them to wash their hands when they're away from home (at school or a friend's house) before eating and after touching anything that might not be sanitary, such as anything in a public bathroom.

Some colds have been known to turn into more serious problems, like sinus infections, bronchitis, or even pneumonia, so it's in your best interest to do everything you can to prevent them. Increase your intake of vitamin C, preferably through real food such as fresh citrus fruit, fresh-squeezed juice, strawberries, and broccoli. Also …

➤ Do lots of *pranayama* to keep your breathing passages clear. Keep a tissue nearby! *Pranayama* techniques also work to increase and strengthen the immune system.

➤ When possible, breathe through your nose instead of your mouth. Your nasal passages are designed to filter out pollutants, viruses, and bacteria. If you are too congested to breathe through your nose, sit with your head over a bowl of hot water and a towel draped over your head to clear that congestion.

➤ If your cold comes with a headache, try the previously mentioned headache re-lief suggestions.

➤ Poses that open the chest can feel great when you are congested. Try the bow, fish, and cobra poses (all in Chapter 14).

Wise Yogi Tells Us

If you have nasal congestion, try using a *neti* pot. A *neti* pot is a pot specifically tailored to the nose! A mixture of saline solution is poured into one nostril and comes out the other nostril with the appropriate tilt of the head. *Neti* pots are traditionally used in the yoga practice of a cleansing ritual called *neti* (described in Chapter 8). Ask your yoga teacher about this specially made little pot which can help to remove nasal irritants and clear nasal passages.

When It's More Serious

Unfortunately, despite our best efforts, sometimes we get very sick. Competent med-ical care is crucial if you have a serious condition, but yoga can help, too. When your body is aligned, strong, and flexible, it will be able to fight off illness more effectively. When your mind is calm, peaceful, and optimistic, your body will be even better at battling the bad stuff. Keep your body filled with *prana* and positive thoughts, and don't give up hope. Hope is the best nurse of all.

Yoga can be excellent for serious conditions, but we recommend practicing one on one with an experienced and knowledgeable yoga teacher if you …

➤ Have recently had surgery.

➤ Are pregnant (take one of the excellent prenatal yoga classes offered in many cities).

Ouch!

This book isn't meant to replace your doctor! If you're sick, injured, or the victim of any kind of chronic pain, seek medical attention from a licensed medical professional. Yoga can be a great complement to your physician's treatment plan. Ask your doctor how yoga fits in!

➤ Have cancer, diabetes, epilepsy, heart disease, high blood pressure, HIV, multiple sclerosis, or any other serious condition.

➤ Have a debilitating physical handicap.

The one-on-one, personal attention to your specific needs can be a tremendous asset to your healing process.

AIDS

Because the AIDS virus attacks the immune system, yoga can be of great benefit in extending life expectancy by encouraging the immune system to rally. Practice your regular yoga routine diligently. The general and gentle nonviolent practice of *Hatha Yoga* will increase your overall circulation and the delivery of oxygen throughout your body. *Pranayama* techniques (Chapter 7) and relaxation techniques (Chapter 19) both boost the immune system.

Arthritis

Chronic joint pain—ncluding such common joint problems as TMJ, tennis elbow, and carpal tunnel syndrome—can be seriously debilitating. If you suffer from arthritis in particular or joint pain in general, relaxation is key to easing your distress. Yoga can be a great help, but if you have arthritis, it's important not to push yourself beyond what your body can do. Don't exercise joints that are inflamed.

However, many people with arthritis drastically decrease activity due to pain. Your joints should periodically be mobilized to keep them limber and clean. Yoga encourages you to keep moving, gently. As long as the following postures don't hurt, include them in your regular practice:

➤ *Vinyasa* routines (Chapter 16), such as a slow sun salutation, are excellent for maintaining your mobility.

➤ Try self-massage to bring warmth and circulation to painful areas.

➤ *Pranayama* (Chapter 7) increases your circulation and helps with pain.

Asthma, Allergies, and Respiratory Problems

When your breath is disturbed, your *prana* delivery system is disturbed, and that's a big deal. You don't want to mess with the life force! If you suffer from asthma, allergies, or other respiratory problems, you know how frustrating, let alone dangerous, breathing difficulties can be. Try the following to keep your breath flowing freely:

➤ Practice poses that open and stretch the chest: tree and warrior poses (Chapter 13, "What Do You Stand For?"); fish, bow, and cobra poses (Chapter 14). Be careful not to hold your breath while holding these poses.

➤ Two deep breaths while holding a pose are better than 10 shallow breaths.

➤ Eat a healthy diet!

Cancer

In 1931, Dr. Otto Heinrich Warburg won the Nobel Prize in Medicine for his discovery that suboptimal oxygenation of tissues and cells is the underlying cause of cancer. Translation? Give your body oxygen! *Yogis* discovered thousands of years ago that the quality of one's breath has a direct and profound influence on the quality of one's life. *Pranayama,* therefore, is one of the best things you can do to keep your body filled with oxygen (and *prana!*).

In addition, evidence is building to support the claim that you can prevent many cancers by changing lifestyle habits like smoking, drinking, and high fat intake. However, knowing this doesn't help the person already afflicted with cancer, and may even make you feel worse. If you have cancer, don't blame yourself or waste time thinking about what you might have done differently. Instead, focus on your future and getting well.

Many cancers are curable, and even advanced cancers have been cured. Several studies have shown that cancer survivors tend to take charge of their illness by learning all they can about it (*svadhyaya*—see Chapter 6, "Walking Yoga's Eightfold Path") and by having a positive attitude. Believe in yourself, the healing power of your body, and the healing power of your treatment regimen. Cultivate your own spirituality. Meditate, fill your lungs and body with *prana* through breathing exercises, and practice your *Hatha Yoga* routine slowly, steadily, and consistently to improve your circulation and overall strength. It is also important to eat a diet consisting of pure, whole foods. Bring meditation into your life. Meditation removes obstacles and illusions (see Chapter 4, "Yoga Mind Power: Go with the Flow").

Cardiovascular Disease

Your heart is the pump that keeps your body running. When your heart begins to lose efficiency or fails, your life is in immediate jeopardy. The best course of action is to prevent heart disease by eating a healthy, low-fat diet and by exercising regularly, but even perfectly healthy individuals are sometimes struck by cardiovascular disease. Maybe it's a matter of genetics. Sometimes the reason is a mystery. The treatment needn't be mysterious, however. In addition to your regular medical care, remember the following:

➤ Yoga can help you make the lifestyle changes you need for a better, happier heart. Yoga will decrease stress and increase circulation.

➤ The fastest way to reduce stress is to alter the breath. Deepen it. Inverted postures (see Chapter 15, "Come on, Body, Let's Do the Twist") take pressure off the heart because it doesn't have to work as hard to pump blood to the extremities. More oxygen is pushed through the wall of the lungs, purifying the blood—but first get your doctor's permission to practice inversions.

➤ Yoga *asanas* in general stretch the major blood vessels, keeping them open and elastic.

Wise Yogi Tells Us

Even if you are unable to do yoga because of illness, injury, or chronic pain, visualizing yourself going through the postures has been known to improve *prana*, the life force. First visualize the pose, then visualize flowing into the pose, becoming one with the pose, flowing out of the pose, and releasing. Like Pavlov's dog, ultimately we can think "fish pose," and our body will receive all the benefits. We are more than our bodies and must learn to work with whatever body we are given.

Diabetes

If you have diabetes, your blood has too much sugar and you may need to take insulin, which reduces blood sugar levels. Diabetes can be extremely serious if it isn't treated, but when treated, people with this condition can live virtually unencumbered by health problems.

For the diabetic, dietary control and weight control are crucial. Yoga is great for both and is, therefore, an excellent addition to the regular routine of anyone with diabetes. Yoga also helps with stress and improves the function of the pancreas, the organ that regulates blood sugar by producing insulin. Include the following in your routine:

➤ Obviously, you'll need a healthy diet. Yoga builds your confidence, concentration, and willpower, enabling you to want to stick with healthy eating habits.

➤ Since circulation in the extremities is important for those with diabetes, try resting your legs up against a wall as you lie back and relax. A slow, steady *vinyasa* routine will also help you maintain good circulation.

➤ Practice *pranayama* (Chapter 7) and meditation to help gain focus and control.

Illness, disease, and pain don't have to keep you from a fulfilling yoga practice. With your doctor's and yoga teacher's guidance, progress at a pace that is right for you and let yoga help your body help itself.

The Least You Need to Know

➤ Your body consists of five bodies: the physical you; the you containing *prana*, the life force; the emotional you; the intellectual you; and the blissful, peaceful you.

➤ The regular practice of yoga *asanas* and *pranayama* exercises is a great way to prevent health problems and to help your body cure itself when health problems occur.

➤ Yoga can help with your minor health complaints, such as colds, minor back pain, and fatigue.

➤ With the approval of your doctor, yoga can also help more serious problems, such as diabetes, cancer, and migraine headaches.

Yoga for Everyone!

You don't exist in a vacuum, of course, so in Part 7, we introduce you to "partner yoga," and then we address your unique needs, strengths, and challenges with information on yoga for women only (from PMS to postpartum depression), yoga for men (trust us, guys, you're gonna love it!), yoga for kids (infants to teens), group yoga (it's a family affair!), and yoga for seniors (the golden years aren't called "golden" for nothing!).

Young or old, girl or guy—a regular yoga practice will enhance and enrich your experiences and your relationships with the people you love.

Chapter 23

Yoga for Two

In This Chapter

➤ How yoga is different when practiced in pairs

➤ Great postures for partners

➤ How yoga can make all your relationships—even the sexual—more spiritual

➤ Meditation for two

Why practice yoga with anyone else? Isn't yoga a solitary and self-reflective pursuit? Yes, it is. But the journey can also involve spiritual communion between two bodies and two souls. Also, postures you can perform alone can be modified or performed more deeply or intensely when someone else helps you. Plus, practicing yoga with a friend, partner, or spouse can deepen your relationship, because you'll be undertaking at least certain legs of your yoga journey hand in hand.

Double Your Insight

Finding wholeness and balance within yourself is important. However, because you probably aren't a hermit living alone in a cave or on a mountaintop, it's also important to find wholeness and balance in your relationships. Practicing yoga with a fellow *yogi* can expand your sense of balance and improve your relationship, not only with your yoga partner but with all your fellow earthlings.

Double yoga helps to unfold your awareness, so it blankets your entire household, community, country, and planet. It gives you insight into the journeys, desires, suffering, and joy of others. It helps you to understand that every human being is as complex, interesting, and beautiful as you are.

Postures for Partners: Part 1

So let's try a few! Grab (nonviolently, of course!) your spouse, partner, child, or friend, and try this set of postures for partners.

Be a Mountain Range

A first and easy posture to try is the mountain pose, but since there are two of you, let's make it a mountain range.

Be a mountain range.

1. Face your partner, standing about two feet apart, and close your eyes. This distance is close enough to allow you to sense each other and to hold hands without arm strain, but far enough away to allow you to maintain a sense of your own space.

2. After you're both centered, hold hands. Take some time to become aware of your partner across from you (keep your eyes closed). Feel your partner's form and energy, then feel the energy flow between you as it traverses the bridge made from your joined hands.

3. Next, connect with the grounding energy of the earth. Feel how it pulls you toward its center. Feel your feet and legs connecting and becoming one with the earth.

4. Let the earth's energy move through your body, from toe to head and beyond, and through your joined hands so that you and your partner are joined with the earth-like mountains.

Warrior 2 Pose for Two

This pose will help you find balance with a partner. In the process, you'll both become stronger.

The warrior 2 pose for two.

1. Stand with one of you in front (Partner A) and one behind (Partner B). Each perform the warrior 2 pose (Chapter 13, "What Do You Stand For?"). Once you are both in position, Partner A balances the extended arms and hands on top of the back of Partner B's extended arms, forming a chain of energy.

2. Partner B keeps Partner A's arms and hands at shoulder height. Partner B will expend more effort, but Partner A should keep the arms energized and strong rather than let them sag limply on partner B's. Partner B should be supporting an energy flow, not a limp noodle.

3. Switch sides. Now Partner A holds Partner B's arms up. Breathe. Try to increase the length of time holding the pose. Encourage each other to hang in there. This pose is difficult and builds arm strength in addition to doubling the warrior energy.

Stretch and Pull

Both partners receive a nice spine stretch in this pose for two.

Stretch and pull.

1. Again, stand with one partner in front (Partner A) and one behind (Partner B). Partner B squats with heels on the floor. Partner A performs a forward bend, keeping the knees straight or slightly bending them and folding the torso forward at the hips. Partner A should be able to see Partner B between his or her legs. (Peek-a-boo!)

2. Partner A reaches both hands between the legs, and Partner B grasps Partner A's wrists, pulling slightly to help Partner A stretch.

3. At the same time, Partner B bends down into a full squat, stretching the back.

4. Hold and take some breaths.

5. Switch places and do it again.

Lengthen Your Spine Together

Continue to lengthen the spine—maybe even grow an inch with this one!

Lengthen your spine together.

1. Face each other, hold hands, then take a big step away from each other.

2. Bend at your hips, but don't clunk heads! Be sure to step far enough away from each other that you don't collide.

3. Bring your tailbones up and out. Take turns pulling gently on each other to lengthen your spines.

4. Then find a balance—pull—and both of you come down into a squat. Keep your heels on the ground. Stretch that spine.

5. Slowly come back up, balancing and stretching all the way back to standing.

The "S" in Sex Stands for "Spirituality"

Practicing yoga with your partner can deepen all aspects of your relationship, even your physical relationship. When practicing "couples yoga" with your partner or spouse, don't simply hold the positions. Take full advantage of your partner's proximity. Feel your partner's energy, body shape, and movement.

Truly connecting with your partner on a spiritual level is a much more blissful experience than mere physical connection. It can even be a bit alarming if you aren't used to really knowing someone on this level, because souls are much more sensitive than bodies. This is a goal you can work toward when practicing yoga with your partner.

Problems in your relationship may surface, too, as you work together in different postures. You should be prepared for this possibility. Your bodies can reflect your minds, so when you have difficulty with a double posture, look into what's wrong and see if you can't find what's happening on a deeper level. Working through the barriers in your physical partnership can reveal the barriers in

Ouch!

When you're helping someone else stretch (or he or she is helping you), keep the lines of communication open. You can't feel when someone else is starting to hurt (unless you're extremely attuned), so let each other know when you're being pushed or pulled just far enough.

A Yoga Minute

Mae West once said, "Sex is an emotion in motion." How true! One of the benefits of the fourth *yama, brahmacharya* (see Chapter 6, "Walking Yoga's Eightfold Path"), is that it teaches you to separate lust from a purer, spiritual connection. When you're fraught with emotional desire for the physical, you cannot perceive a deeper reality. Transcending intense emotions permits the spirit to manifest itself.

your spiritual partnership. Take the lessons you learn about each other into your hearts and memorize them. They're lessons in true love!

Postures for Partners: Part 2

Double yoga is a fun way to exercise your relationships. Let's try a few more poses for two.

Massage Your Spines Together

This pose will help your partner connect to the muscles alongside the spine. A flexible spine equals a youthful body. Help your partner loosen up his or her spine.

Massage your spines together.

Ouch!

Be sensitive to your partner's limits when practicing any partner pose.

1. Partner A sits in the child's pose (see Chapter 18, "Take the Forward Path").

2. Partner B stands behind Partner A and places a palm on either side of Partner A's spine at the lower back. Partner B gradually walks the hands up to the neck and back down to the lower back. Partner B keeps as much of the palm on Partner A's back as possible at all times, pressing gently. Don't press directly on the spine; stay on either side.

Forward Bend Together

This pose starts to look complicated, but it really isn't. It's only two poses in one. Partner B helps Partner A lengthen the spine by pushing down on Partner A's hipbone. Conversely, Partner A helps Partner B lengthen the hamstrings by pushing down on Partner B's heels.

Forward bend together.

1. Partner A gets into the child's pose with arms outstretched in front (Chapter 18).

2. Partner B stands in front of Partner A. Partner A holds Partner B's ankles as Partner B assumes the downward facing dog posture (Chapter 18) over the top of Partner A, placing the hands on either side of Partner A's hips, palms facing in.

3. Partner B helps Partner A lengthen the spine, while Partner A helps Partner B lengthen the hamstrings.

4. Hold as long as is comfortable, then switch positions.

Forward Bend and Backbend Together

Try this one with a partner who is about the same size as you are. If one of you is much larger, he or she should be Partner A, and the positions shouldn't be reversed.

1. Partner A sits on the floor a few feet from a wall with the back to the wall and the feet in front and together. Bending at the waist, Partner A brings the chest toward the thighs. Bend your knees if needed.

2. Partner B lies on Partner A's back, facing up, and props the feet against the wall so that the feet are slightly higher than the head. Partner B's fingers can rest lightly on the ground on either side of Partner A's hips.

3. Hold for a while, then switch.

Forward bend and back-bend together.

Boat Pose for Two

Boat pose for two helps to calm the rocky waters and strengthens tummies, too (or two!).

Boat pose for two.

1. Face each other so that your hips are three to four feet apart. Both partners assume the boat pose (Chapter 18).

2. Place your feet sole to sole, and grasp hands on the outsides of your legs. Now you look like a schooner!

Wise Yogi Tells Us

Try double heart gazing to connect your heart *chakras*. Sit facing each other in any meditative pose with your knees touching. Look into each other's eyes. Really look, past the surface. Place your right hand on your partner's heart, and have your partner place his or her right hand on your heart. Then each partner covers his or her own heart (and the partner's right hand) with the left hand. Feel the energy flowing between your heart *chakras*, connecting you to each other. Close your eyes and continue to feel the energy.

Don't miss out on the great physical, emotional, and spiritual benefits of yoga for two. This type of workout is completely different from solo yoga and can be very fulfilling (although it isn't meant to replace a strong and steady personal *Hatha Yoga* practice). Vary your solitary communion with one of fellowship now and then. Partner yoga will increase your joy.

The Least You Need to Know

➤ Practicing yoga with a partner is fun and can deepen your relationship, including your sexual relationship.

➤ Practicing yoga with a partner can help you stretch farther than you could alone.

➤ Yoga with your partner or spouse can make all aspects of your partnership—physical, emotional, and intellectual—more spiritual.

Chapter 24

For Women Only

In This Chapter

➤ What is beauty?

➤ How yoga can help you through PMS and menstruation

➤ Pregnancy and new motherhood yoga

➤ Yoga for menopause

This chapter is for all you female *yogis* (*yoginis*) out there! Being a woman means certain things biologically and certain things culturally, too. We experience menstruation as our first rite of passage into womanhood, many of us experience childbirth, and eventually we experience menopause. We're also raised in a culture obsessed with beauty, youth, and the female body. Women have many unique challenges, and yoga can help with all of them by helping to keep us fit, strong, clear-thinking, and joyful.

The Truth About Beauty

Beauty really isn't skin-deep. In fact, it has nothing to do with your skin—not really. Beauty begins much deeper, so it's no wonder that many beautiful women don't believe they're beautiful. If you haven't found your inner self and aren't in touch with who you are, you won't be able to perceive your true beauty, even if you just signed a modeling contract. Your inner beauty has nothing to do with your hair color or facial wrinkles or cellulite or breast size. These are transitory features of your soul's container. These aren't you.

The most important first step any woman can take in dealing with the issue of beauty is to practice *ahimsa*, or nonviolence. Nonviolent acceptance of yourself, not only physically but mentally and spiritually, too, is yoga's dictum. Don't commit violence to your body, either physically, by trying to force it to conform to some cultural ideal, or mentally, by hating it or obsessing over it. Remember that your body is a tool. Keep it well maintained so it doesn't interfere with the real you. Keep it clean, strong, and flexible, but also keep it in its place.

The true you is much deeper, more complex, and more spectacular than your body. You're a manifestation of the universe. Finding yourself through yoga means finding the beautiful, spiritual you and bringing it out for everyone to see. Loving yourself means loving the universe, and loving the universe means loving yourself, because you're one and the same: You're both exquisitely radiant.

Kiss PMS Good-Bye

When you're suffering from PMS, you probably don't feel very radiant. PMS, or pre-menstrual syndrome, is a condition that affects a lot of women before the onset of their menstrual periods. Symptoms are as diverse as overall discomfort, bloating, backache, headache, irritability, food cravings, depression, acne, painful or swollen breasts, insomnia, fatigue, even uncharacteristically violent or suicidal behavior. Many women get a little emotional, uncomfortable, and hungrier, but everyone is different, and each woman may experience different symptoms from month to month. Some women experience no symptoms at all.

PMS commonly occurs during the week or two before the start of your period and can last until menstruation starts. Symptoms are generally attributed to the production of hormones related to the menstrual cycle. You may not care about the cause so much as a good remedy when you're in the throes.

How can yoga help? Be dedicated to your regular yoga routine during PMS. Your hormone-wracked body will appreciate the familiar routine and the exercise. The triangle pose (see Chapter 13, "What Do You Stand For?"), sitting poses to open the hips, and twisting poses for lower back stiffness are all excellent for PMS. Although all the *asanas* activate the body, poses that stimulate the glandular and reproductive systems are good to practice during PMS, such as the cobra, bow (both in Chapter 14, "Bending Over Back-bends"), and bridge (Chapter 15, "Come on, Body, Let's Do the Twist") poses.

Wise Yogi Tells Us

When you're feeling particularly PMS-y, lie on your back with your buttocks against a wall. Put your legs up against the wall, separate them a bit, and lie there for a while—very relaxing.

Also, step up your *pranayama* practice (Chapter 7, "Can You Breathe?"). As your body sheds its uterine lining, support it by cleansing the rest of your body through *pranayama* (deep-breathing exercises). *Pranayama* also eases irritability, depression, and moodiness. *Mantra* work, too, can be of great benefit when your emotions are changing rapidly (see Chapter 3, "How Comfortable Are You in Your

Body?"). The steady flow and vibration of a *mantra* soothes your nervous system and can help transform negative outbursts into outbursts of pure inspiration!

Wise Yogi Tells Us

Herbs known to help relieve the symptoms of PMS, such as bloating, pain, and depression, are evening primrose oil, dong quai, blessed thistle, cayenne, raspberry leaves, sarsaparilla, and Siberian ginseng. Look for these herbs in your local health food store, and take as directed. Recent studies show that increased calcium intake can also help relieve the uncomfortable symptoms of PMS.

And no matter how bad PMS is, stress only makes it worse—just one more reason to keep practicing yoga! All of the stress reduction yoga performs on the human body can also help to lessen the effects of PMS. Don't forget *shavasana* (the relaxation pose in Chapter 19, "Dead to the World")—do it as often as you can. When you are feeling physically or emotionally uncomfortable, you'll welcome *shavasana's* utterly relaxed state, especially when you get so relaxed that you don't even feel your body anymore!

Meditation, too, can be helpful when you are uncomfortable but in a good frame of mind. Meditation, including *shavasana,* can help you move beyond your physical body for a while, to give yourself a break from the aches and pains.

Going Full Cycle: Celebrating Menstruation

Some women are pleased by the arrival of their menstrual period each month—or so we hear. Most of us are a little miffed. "*This* again?" we think. "Why do I have to go through this every month!" Do you really want to know?

Technically speaking, menstruation is part of your body's fertility cycle. About every month, from puberty to menopause, your womb first builds up nourishment for a potential embryo and, after ovulation, if pregnancy has not occurred, sheds this tissue in a self-cleansing process before beginning to prepare anew for next month's cycle. All of this happens due to the work of your hormones, which fluctuate throughout the month but seem to cause the most trouble in terms of discomfort during the premenstrual period.

Ouch!

PMS can literally be a big pain, and eating certain foods just before you expect PMS symptoms can make it worse. Even if you crave them, try to avoid chocolate, anything with caffeine, alcohol, excess salt, red meat, sugar, and overly processed foods, which seem to aggravate PMS symptoms in some women. Focus on calcium and fiber instead. A fresh apple and a glass of milk, anyone?

But that's not really what you mean when you wonder why you have to go through menstruation—we know that. We're just trying to remind you what it's all about. Your menstrual cycle sets you apart as a woman. (Well, it isn't the *only* clue, but it's certainly an unmistakable clue!) Menstruation is a monthly marker of your fertility and one of the few biologically imposed rituals we have.

Women have often been compared to the moon, probably because both operate in cycles. Study the moon for a few months, watching it nightly as its lighted section swells, then shrinks each month. Feel a kinship with the moon. See if you can notice its effect on you. Do you feel different during a full moon than during a new moon? How does your menstrual cycle synchronize with the moon's cycle? Pay attention to the beautiful regularity of the moon's waxing and waning, then carry that reverence over to your own body. Your cycle is similarly splendid—even if it doesn't always feel that way.

Wise Yogi Tells Us

Rather than fighting gravity, yoga makes a friend of gravity. So during those times when we want to encourage movement out of the body, such as during menstruation, it's counterproductive to work against gravity by practicing inversions like the headstand or the plough (Chapter 15). Thank gravity for helping your body with its monthly "out with the old, in with the new" process and stay right-side up during menstruation.

Incorporating yoga into your menstrual ritual is a nice way to make the experience even more positive. You can do any yoga posture you normally do (except for inversions—skip the headstand and shoulderstand during this week), but you might enjoy creating a special yoga routine for the week of your menstrual period. Try the following variations of poses for your menstrual cycle sessions.

An extra-long *shavasana* (Chapter 19) is the perfect way to end your yoga practice during your menstrual cycle.

You may also want to experiment with the triangle (Chapter 13), the cobra (Chapter 14), the bow (great for cramps if you're up to it, Chapter 14), the wheel (also great for cramps, Chapter 14), the bridge (Chapter 15), the butterfly, the lotus (both in Chapter 17, "Are You Sitting Down?"), and the moon salutation (Chapter 16, "A Continuous Flow") poses. These are all just suggestions to help make this cycle a comfortable one.

A modified child's pose to ease menstruation or bring comfort during pregnancy.

1. Sit in the hero pose, butterfly pose, or lotus pose (all in Chapter 17). Place a few pillows stacked on top of each other directly behind you. Lie back on top of the pillows. Extend your arms over your head. This position opens the Venus *chakra* and is also a good variation to perform during pregnancy.

2. Sit with your feet in front of you, widely separated. Place a few pillows stacked on top of each other in front of your navel. Bend forward, bringing your hands toward your feet.

So, You're Having a Baby!

Pregnancy yoga is slightly different than regular yoga, and perhaps even more wonderful. Yoga helps you develop a greater awareness of your body so you can respond better to your body's subtle signals (such as, "You're doing too much today" or "You need to get up and move today" or "You could really use a hearty serving of broccoli today").

Because yoga gets you moving, you'll be in better shape for the hard work of labor. Recovery and getting back to your prepregnancy shape will be easier, too. Taking a prenatal yoga class can be a lot of fun. You'll get to meet similarly minded pregnant women, you'll get qualified instruction on the safest and most beneficial yoga poses, and you may be more motivated to keep up your workout. Plus, in the last month or two when baby is getting big, he or she may be able to move more freely as you open your body in a stretch.

A few caveats are in order first, however. Take these precautions when practicing pregnancy yoga:

➤ Tell your doctor you are practicing yoga, and get permission for all poses you plan on practicing. If your doctor isn't familiar with yoga, bring pictures of the poses you'd like to do.

➤ Avoid extreme stretching positions and any position that puts pressure on or contracts your uterus. Skull-shining breath may be too jarring for baby, and full forward bends will probably be uncomfortable for you and baby, too.

➤ Avoid full backbends such as wheel pose and full forward bends such as head-to-knee poses—maintain that abdominal space. Give that little him or her a little room in there!

➤ Keep standing poses to a minimum, and never jump into them.

➤ Remember that your center of balance is completely different than it was. Be careful doing balance poses. If you fall, the baby is well-cushioned in your uterus, but you could injure yourself.

➤ Don't lie on your stomach for any pose.

➤ After the twentieth week, don't lie on your back for any pose (which will probably start to become uncomfortable, anyway). The weight of the baby can hinder your blood flow.

Wise Yogi Tells Us

After the twentieth week, practice *shavasana* with lots of pillows, lying on your left side instead of your back.

The following are suggestions only. If any pose feels uncomfortable or strenuous, stop at once. If you experience dizziness, sudden swelling, extreme shortness of breath, or vaginal bleeding, see your doctor immediately. Your best approach to these postures is to listen to your body and to never take it where it doesn't want to go.

➤ *Tadasana,* **mountain pose (Chapter 13).** Focus on tilting your lower back in to prevent the weight of the baby from pressing against your lumbar. Bend your knees slightly and place your hands on top of your knees. Tighten your thigh muscles and watch your kneecaps lift up. Straighten your legs and try to lift your kneecaps.

The added weight of pregnancy can create a condition called "lordosis," a swayback effect. Practice tadasana, the mountain pose, and concentrate on maintaining the proper spinal and pelvic alignment.

➤ *Shavasana,* **corpse pose (Chapter 19).** After your twentieth week, practice *shavasana* lying on your left side. A pillow for your head and pillows between your knees can take pressure of your neck, lower back, and hips, which may all be suffering from the change in your center of gravity.

After the twentieth week of pregnancy, practice shavasana *by lying on your left side.*

➤ **Hero pose (Chapter 17).** Sitting in this pose helps to reduce swelling in your ankles, reduces fatigue, and improves circulation in your legs. Place a stack of pillows behind you and lean back. Bring your hands alongside your body to push yourself back up.

➤ **Child's pose (Chapter 18, "Take the Forward Path").** Support your body with a stack of pillows placed between your knees, or stand on your knees and cross your arms over the back of a chair and lean forward. You might want a pillow or blanket under your knees as well, to protect and cushion them.

A variation of the child's pose during pregnancy.

Ouch!

At the first sign of leg cramps (common in pregnancy), draw your toes upward and push out your heel. Practice this movement so you can be ready to perform it in a split second when a leg cramp wakes you up in the middle of the night.

➤ **Simple hamstring stretches.** Your hamstrings are the tendons at the back of your knee. Hamstring stretches relieve pressure on your lower back. Be gentle when you stretch.

➤ **Twisting poses should be performed gently.** When not pregnant, the focus should be on twisting the entire spine. During pregnancy, however, most of your twisting will be in your neck, shoulders, and head. Lift your spine as you inhale, twist as you exhale.

➤ **Use chairs for support whenever you can.** For example, try the warrior 2 pose or side angle stretch (Chapter 13) seated on the center of a chair. It is more freeing and takes the weight off your legs.

The side angle stretch variation during pregnancy.

➤ **Another way to use a chair is to try the downward facing dog while standing and using the back of the chair for support.** What a wonderful stretch and release for the spine! Holding on to the chair takes some of the pressure off the legs in this pose. You'll feel freer, and so will your little passenger.

The downward facing dog variation during pregnancy. If you don't have a steady, firm chair to use, place your hands against a wall and stretch this way.

➤ **Learn some inspirational *mantras* to practice during childbirth.** They'll be much more productive than yelling and swearing at your partner, midwife, or doctor. Let your baby experience the transcendent vibrations of a *mantra*. If nothing else, transform your "AAAAHHHHHHH!" into "AAAAUUUUMMMM!"

➤ **The butterfly pose can help you relax, open your hips, and prepare for labor.** If your hip joints are tight, sit supported with a pillow under each knee. Hold the position only as long as it is comfortable. Move into an easy pose and rest if you need to.

287

If the butterfly pose is comfortable for you, you might want to try this more advanced squatting pose. Stack the pillows as high on the floor as you need to, to reduce stress on your joints and muscles. When you are ready, return to a seated meditative position and breathe deeply and fully.

New Mama Yoga

Once you're home with your new little bundle, you may be a bit incredulous that you could have any time for yoga. You don't even have time to sleep! The first few weeks of transition are stressful, but also joyful. You may feel alternately ecstatic and despairing, frustrated and overflowing with love.

Practicing yoga now is important because you need the energy. Filling your body with *prana* through breathing exercises and 10 minutes daily in *shavasana* will recharge you and make the little sleep you do get more productive. Your body also needs all its resources to heal itself after childbirth.

You probably need some mental maintenance, too. Your hormones may be making you extra emotional or a little depressed right after childbirth. Add to that the fact that your entire life has changed and will never be the same. Pile on top of that the fact that your jeans look hopelessly small, and even though you aren't pregnant anymore, all you may be able to wear are your old maternity clothes. Remember that it takes time to adjust to any major life change. It will also take your body time to readjust to a nonpregnant state. Be patient. Be kind to yourself. It took you nine months to get to childbirth, so give yourself nine months to get back. You have just accomplished something magnificent, and it has changed you. Accept the change lovingly and with joy.

Give yourself time to practice yoga each day, either when your baby is sleeping or when your partner, a family member, or a friend can play with the baby. Consider it pampering time and a well-deserved reward.

With your doctor's approval, you can usually start gentle yoga postures two weeks after delivery, a few weeks longer if you had a cesarean section. Hold off on inverted poses for at least six weeks.

All women have postnatal bleeding for a few weeks after pregnancy. Watch this flow for signs that you're going too fast. If the bleeding gets heavier or brighter red, you need to slow down and give your doctor a call. Start with just a few poses, and gradually work back to your regular routine as your body lets you know it's ready.

The most beneficial pose for you right now is *shavasana* (Chapter 19), which you can even do on the day you give birth. *Shavasana* can help ease labor pains. It can help you recoup your energy before all that pushing! It can also help you to relax after the whole process is finished and you have a sleeping baby on your chest.

Any chance you get, take some deep breaths and practice these revitalizing poses. You'll handle all your new challenges with greater inner strength and energy. The following poses are also wonderful for a gentle postpregnancy routine:

Wise Yogi Tells Us

A high-sugar diet will make you feel tired any time, but especially in the early weeks after childbirth. Sure, you deserve a treat now and then, but a diet based on whole-grain foods like whole-wheat bread and brown rice, sufficient iron (best sources are dark, leafy greens, wheat germ, and meat), and lots of vegetables is the best diet to combat fatigue.

➤ *Tadasana,* **the mountain pose (Chapter 13).** Take some time to stand in the mountain pose, and notice how your center of gravity has shifted yet again. Let *tadasana* help you reacquaint yourself with your newly autonomous body.

➤ **The butterfly pose (Chapter 17).** Place pillows under your knees. Notice how this pose feels different than it did when you were pregnant.

➤ **Child's pose (Chapter 18).** Let yourself be the child for a few minutes each day.

More important than any postures at this point is your attitude. Being a new mother isn't easy. If you're feeling frustrated or unhappy and think you must be a bad mother, give yourself a break! All new mothers feel like that sometimes. Remember *ahimsa:* Treat yourself nonviolently. Your feelings

Wise Yogi Tells Us

The postpartum (the period after childbirth) time is a good time to read the *Yoga Sutra* or other yoga texts. Keep them on a bedside table or end table to read while nursing your baby or while baby is sleeping.

are completely normal. Don't be afraid to talk to your partner, your close friends, or a counselor about your feelings. Just remember that you're entering an exciting new leg of your life journey.

Easing Through Menopause

Menopause is the time of life when a woman stops ovulating. Although the age at which it occurs varies greatly, it commonly occurs around age 50. Yet menopause means much more to women than this simple biological definition. The thought of menopause is daunting to many, and it's no wonder! Our culture puts so much emphasis on youth and beauty, especially for women, that aging is difficult enough.

Because women are finally beginning to share their experiences of menopause, and more information is available, this transition from fertility to the next stage of life is easier to prepare for. Far from being the end of life, menopause signals a period of life during which spiritual growth can soar. Women who have passed through menopause often feel stronger, more in charge of their lives, and more intimately acquainted with their souls than ever before. Age brings wisdom, and once a woman is no longer a childbearer, her body can focus on its own journey. Increasing numbers of strong, vibrant, amazing older women have become important figures in our culture. Look to these women as examples for your own life. This next stage of your journey may be the most thrilling yet. It's certainly full of possibilities.

But first, you have to get through the menopause, and that isn't always pleasant. A hot flash is still a hot flash (you could call it a recharge!), whether or not it signals an exhilarating life transition. Menopause comes with lots of other physical complaints beyond the often-cited hot flashes. Dizziness, depression, heart palpitations, decreased sex drive, and shortness of breath are all symptoms of decreased estrogen levels.

Yoga balances the endocrine system and can ease the difficult transition by stabilizing hormone levels. Inverted postures are particularly helpful for hot flashes, because they cool the body and fill it with *prana*. *Pranayama*, too, is cooling to the body.

As you work through menopause, incorporate these postures into your yoga routine:

➤ The headstand and other inversions, like the shoulderstand and plough (all in Chapter 15). If you've never mastered the headstand, now's the time to try. The headstand may reduce your hot flashes. All the inversions will make you feel more vital, too, because they replenish and rejuvenate your body.

Ouch!

When we hear the word *menopause*, most of us think of hot flashes, but you can experience a range of other physical symptoms. Considering menopause can last for five years, you'll probably want to do everything you can to minimize the unpleasantness.

➤ Downward facing dog and other forward-bending postures, such as standing head to knees and *yoga mudra* (all in Chapter 18). These forward-bending poses help you focus inwardly, an important process right now. Instead of shunning your body or feeling that it has betrayed you, embrace it, get to know it all over again, and let it work for you, leading you to a higher spiritual plane.

➤ Sun salutation (Chapter 16). Celebrate how your body has moved beyond moonlike cycles and catapulted like a rocket on toward the sun. Make the sun your newest ally. If you're up to it, start rising at dawn to practice yoga. Notice how, although the earth moves and turns and changes, the sun burns steadily and luminously in the center of our solar system. Meditate on how your body has become sunlike and strong, glowing with newfound steadiness and bliss.

➤ Any weight-bearing postures and activities. A drop in your estrogen level can cause you to lose bone mass, but you can easily counter this by exercising your bones. Postures that put stress on your bones, such as inversions, standing postures, and downward facing dog, all increase bone mass. Light weight lifting is great for your bones, and so is walking. Take a walk in the fresh air every day to keep your bones strong, your lungs full, and your heart light.

➤ Place a folded blanket or pillows about nine inches high against a wall. Support your lower and midback on the blanket, stretch your legs up the wall, and let your shoulder blades and head rest on the floor. Rest in this pose for 10 minutes with your eyes closed; focus on your breathing. This pose is cooling and therapeutic for any pelvic or abdominal problems.

➤ Start regular meditation. You're in an excellent time of life to begin meditation. You have a better sense of yourself than ever before. Take advantage of your wisdom and experience, and reap the benefits of meditation.

Most important, know that your life is far from over. You're a strong, vibrant woman with much to offer the world. Cultivate your soul like a garden and find your place in the universe.

The Least You Need to Know

➤ Beauty has nothing to do with your physical appearance. If you care for your body and radiate inner bliss, you'll be beautiful.

➤ Yoga can help reduce symptoms of PMS and menstruation.

➤ Yoga can be tailored to accommodate pregnancy and new motherhood.

➤ Yoga can ease the transition of menopause.

Chapter 25

Yoga for the Whole Family

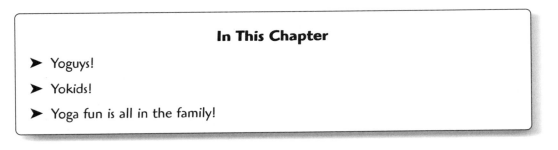

In This Chapter

➤ Yoguys!

➤ Yokids!

➤ Yoga fun is all in the family!

Don't worry, we haven't forgotten the rest of you who don't happen to be women between adolescence and the golden years. People of all ages and both sexes can be *yogis*, and each group has its unique characteristics and problems. If the "For Women Only" chapter didn't happen to be directed at you, we hope you'll feel not only included but warmly welcomed in this chapter.

This chapter includes yoga adventures for all members of the family—the whole clan! Whether you practice yoga individually or together, it is an invaluable way to bring all family members—girls, guys, moms, dads, kids, whoever makes up the family you love—peace, health, and joy.

Mucho Macho

This section is for all you guys out there. Sure, we know lots of you have enrolled in yoga classes, and lots more are wondering what it's all about. Lots more of you, however, are probably just a little suspicious. We hope that so far, many of your questions have been answered, but here are a few more things to think about—you know ... *guy stuff.*

Isn't Yoga for "Chicks"?

Maybe you've picked up this book because yoga interests you, but you just aren't sure yoga is a "guy thing." Isn't it sort of like home economics class or going to the ballet? Granted, if you took a survey today, you would probably find that in any given city,

there are more women taking yoga classes than men. For some reason, women seem to be more comfortable taking exercise classes. But the imbalance is quickly shifting. Why should women get all the fitness benefits of yoga? And why should men miss out on the camaraderie and guided instruction of a class? And why should *anyone* miss out on the mental clarity and inner peace yoga can offer?

A Yoga Minute

Although yoga originated long before recorded history (so there's no telling whose *idea* it actually was), men were certainly instrumental in its refinement and philosophical evolution.

Many men throughout history have devoted their lives to becoming sagacious *yogis*, and today, many of the major schools of yoga—Iyengar Yoga, Sivananda Yoga, Bikram's Yoga—were started by men. So why not practice yoga? It can only make you healthier, stronger, and more flexible. The next time that important woman in your life suggests that you ought to get into yoga, give it a try!

Where's the Team?

You guys who've left that locker-room attitude back in high school gym class can skip ahead to the flexibility section. But let's face it: A lot of guys are very comfortable being athletic in a team situation. Football teams, basketball teams, baseball teams, hockey teams, soccer teams—these are all familiar scenarios for the average American guy. Two teams compete, and one of them wins. No wonder yoga seems a little strange and unfamiliar. No team, no points, no scoring method … and no winner is proclaimed and carried around on everyone's shoulders. Heck, there isn't even a coach on the sidelines you can pour your cooler of water over when the workout is done!

Or so it would seem. Think of it this way: You and everyone else in your yoga class, or your circle of friends and family, or even the world, are a team. You're all seeking a common goal: fitness, happiness, and eventually, self-actualization.

Who's the other team? Let's rephrase that: *What's* the other team? The other team is a surly bunch of characters: self-doubt, negative thoughts, jealousy, hate, violence, illness, pain, and suffering. Formidable opponents! But your team can beat them, and it's up to you to set an example for your team members. Follow yoga's principles, practice the exercises, learn deep breathing, even try meditation. You'll be learning about yourself and learning how to live in the world, too, which is really the same as learning how to be a great team player.

And if you are a yoga dad, yoga can enhance the most important team in your life— your family.

But How Do You Win?

Best of all, with yoga, everybody wins. No, that's not some sappy cop-out. One of the most difficult things for some men to accept about yoga is the idea of noncompeti- tiveness. Yoga has nothing to do with one-upmanship, so it would be against yoga's principles to say that the achievement of each new posture is another "point" for you. On the other hand, the achievement of each new posture *is* like a point against the other team—the suffering, illusion, and illness team. If you can see yoga as a competition against negativity rather than a competition against another person (be- cause that would be like competing with your own team members), then maybe you can fit your competitive nature comfortably into yoga after all.

Although you may not be one of them, some men (and women, and kids) get dis- couraged easily when they aren't immediately skilled at an activity. If yoga is difficult for you at first, the hardest part of all may be adjusting your thinking. Don't compare yourself to anyone else. Even though you're on the same "team" as your fellow *yogis,* in another sense, you are alone in your journey. Only you can determine what your body can do now and what it will be able to do after further progress. Don't punish yourself or criticize yourself for being unable to accomplish an exercise. Cultivate pa- tience with yourself and your body, and your body will respond in ways you never thought it could.

And when your workout is over, especially if it's a hot summer day, why not pull out all the stops, fill up a bucket with water, and pour it over your own head! You deserve it!

These Muscles Don't Stretch

Another problem men commonly have with yoga is their lack of flexibility. From an early age, men are often encouraged to gain strength, but strength without stretching causes muscles to shorten, even if they gain bulk. The strongest man in the world may not be able to touch his toes.

"But the strongest man in the world looks great!" you may protest. "And who needs to touch his toes, anyway?" Flexibility is important for men for several reasons:

➤ Flexible bodies are most resistant to injury. Tendons and muscles become more elastic and can bend farther without tearing.

➤ Getting up in the morning is a lot easier, and your body is less stiff when you have good flexibility.

➤ Adding flexibility to your workout gives you a three-pronged approach to physi- cal fitness: strength training, cardiovascular training, and flexibility training.

This approach is more holistic, developing all aspects of your physical body and maintaining a healthier balance.

➤ If you're ever forced to sit on the floor for a long period of time, you won't mind as much.

➤ A flexible body encourages a flexible mind.

➤ Flexibility can make sex a lot more fun! (Isn't *that* reason enough all by itself?)

Just remember that yoga can do great things for your health and your life. The exercises will tone and strengthen your body in ways that are both different and complementary to your other physical activities. Or if you're sedentary, yoga is a great way to move into a physical lifestyle. Yoga's deep-breathing exercises and meditation can also be new ways for you to discover the limitless possibilities of your body and mind. Give it a try—and welcome to the team!

A Yoga Minute

The following are two styles of yoga for yoguys (and yogals!) who are looking for physical challenges:

➤ **Ashtanga Yoga** literally means the "Eight Limbs of Yoga," as defined by Patanjali in his *Yoga Sutra*. However, it has come to be seen in our society as a *Hatha Yoga* practice that includes an intense *vinyasa* workout (see Chapter 16, "A Continuous Flow").

➤ **Power Yoga** (see *The Complete Idiot's Guide to Power Yoga* and Beryl Bender Birch's book, *Power Yoga*) is a specific, highly athletic form of yoga that is based on the Western conception of *Ashtanga Yoga*. It includes high-intensity, choreographed sequences of postures combined with breath and is quite popular among athletes and others seeking a physically demanding workout.

Here are some good yoga exercises for yoguys:

➤ Those who require cardiovascular exertion. Look for Power Yoga or *Ashtanga* classes in your area, or invent some challenging *vinyasa* for yourself (see Chapter 16).

➤ Sitting postures that increase flexibility in the legs and hips, such as the hero and butterfly pose (see Chapter 17, "Are You Sitting Down?").

➤ Standing postures to increase your confidence when it seems like you can't get your body to do anything, such as the mountain; warrior 1, 2, and 3; and lightning bolt (see Chapter 13, "What Do You Stand For?").

➤ Inversions to replenish and balance your entire body, such as the bridge, shoulderstand, headstand, and handstand (see Chapter 15, "Come on, Body, Let's Do the Twist").

➤ *Shavasana* (see Chapter 19, "Dead to the World"). The corpse pose may be incredibly challenging for you, because ironically, it *isn't* challenging! (Well, not in the typical sense.) Practicing *shavasana* may be the one time in your day when you can completely release challenges and simply "be." Completely relaxing your body and mind isn't as easy as it sounds. Even if you love a good challenge, remember that you need to maintain inner balance. Life isn't always challenging, nor should it be. Maybe you yearn for a space in your life without challenges. *Shavasana*—indeed, all of yoga—can be that space.

➤ Any others that look interesting or fun to you!

And gentlemen, no matter how self-sufficient you are, consider taking a yoga class, because a yoga class is a place where you can go just for yourself. A lot of men are used to exercising in groups, but yoga lets you move, breath, and think without reference to anyone else. Taking a class will give your practice structure, plus the chance to really learn about yourself—not in terms of how others see you, but in terms of who you really are.

Spirituality: Not a Matter of Gender

Remember yoga's traditional, ultimate purpose? Yoga was designed to help discipline the body so it doesn't get in the way of the mind. Meditation can be an important part of a yoga journey, but even if you don't sit for 20 minutes a day chanting "*Om,*" you can still live your life in a more spiritual manner.

But do you want to live more spiritually? What does "spiritual" mean for guys? The same thing it means for anyone! Life is mysterious, beautiful, sometimes sorrowful, sometimes joyful. Bad things happen, good things happen—or at least, things happen we tend to label "bad" or "good." No matter who you are or what gender you happen to be, yoga encourages you to embrace your life and live it with respect, reverence, contentment, and in harmony with everyone and everything else on the planet.

So remember, guys: Yoga isn't just about exercise, although it can really enhance your physical life. Yoga is about the whole you. Women may tend to talk about emotional issues more, but that doesn't mean guys don't think about the big questions. Yes, we're on to you! And some of you, we know, are very interested in talking about the things that make life worth living: What is truth, how can I find meaning, how can I be a better person, how can I improve the world, how can I nurture joy and happiness within myself, among my friends, within my family?

A Yoga Minute

In his book *Sacred Sexuality*, Georg Feuerstein writes:

"Today, adventurers of the spirit who boldly scale the mountain of self-discipline and self-transcendence are as good as extinct. We have too limited a view of our humanness; hence we also have too limited a view of our own sexuality. Yet we cannot live fully as sexual–erotic beings without first recovering our spiritual depth. Our sexuality can help us get in touch again with that depth; it can serve as a gateway to the spiritual dimension."

It all comes down to balance. If you tend to be a physical kind of guy, great! But don't neglect your mind, your feelings, and your spiritual search for self-knowledge and universal truth. And if you are the cerebral type or the emotional type or the philosophical type who sits around thinking about truth quite a bit and struggling to find it in your own life, great! But don't neglect the needs and potential of your physical self, which can be optimized through a vigorous *Hatha Yoga* practice.

Guys, we are all sentient beings, and when you step way back and look at the big picture, none of us is all that different. In fact, we're all beautifully similar, even as we retain our individuality. Each and every one of us is worth becoming the best whole self we can be. Respect and honor your own path, and the paths of others, and you'll be on your way to fulfilling your greatest potential.

Yokids

Kids take naturally to yoga because it's so much fun. Getting the whole family involved in a yoga routine is a great way to keep you motivated. When your whole family practices yoga together, the family bond is strengthened. Everyone learns more about the other family members—what they can and can't do, what they like and dislike, how they like to play. Love is built on intimacy like this, and yoga offers the perfect environment to cultivate and nurture family intimacy.

Turn Off the TV and Play!

Kids today watch a lot of television and play a lot of video games. Sure, some television is stimulating and offers children valuable information. But healthy kids are built from exercise, nutritious food, and imaginative play. Encourage your kids to turn off the tube and get moving, using both their bodies and their minds more actively. Interacting with you and with each other (other siblings or friends) builds children's social skills and teaches them much more about the world than any half-hour sitcom or 60-minute talk show.

The Lessons Yoga Teaches Kids

Yoga teaches kids valuable lessons about life. You'll probably teach your children all of the following in one way or another, but yoga can deepen and reinforce all of these healthy and life-affirming ideas:

➤ Exercise is fun!

➤ Exercise equals Active Play.

➤ When the body and the mind combine into imagination, there are no limits.

➤ Things that are good for you don't have to be unpleasant—they can actually be the highlights of your day!

➤ "Feeling" like different animals and objects such as trees makes children more sensitive, not only to their own bodies, but to all our fellow inhabitants of the earth.

➤ Families that play together understand each other better.

➤ The earth and all its creatures have a lot to teach us about how to move and how to live.

➤ Sometimes it's fun to be quiet, still, and reflective.

➤ Kids can learn to be patient, too.

➤ Your body is your friend, ally, and instrument.

Yoga for All Ages and Stages

Yoga is both fun and beneficial for kids of any age. You can do yoga with your newborn infant, your toddler, your preschooler, your kindergartner, your fourth-grader, your eighth-grader, your high school sophomore, your high school graduate. Older kids often enjoy establishing and growing in an individual yoga practice, too. If you've set them on the yoga path, chances are they'll continue it on their own. What a great gift to give your child!

But yoga is a little different, depending on the age of your child. Infant yoga is, naturally, a completely different kind of practice than yoga for teens. In general, encourage younger kids to talk, respond, and flex their imaginations while practicing yoga (except during meditation, which should be quiet and focused for all). Teens may appreciate a more internalized practice, or maybe not, if they are practicing yoga with a group of friends.

Let's look briefly at some yoga approaches for kids of all ages. Also feel free to adapt any of the basic poses in this book in ways that are fun (and safe) for your child's developmental level. For a whole book on yoga for kids, check out *The Complete Idiot's Guide to Yoga with Kids* by Jodi B. Komitor and Eve Adamson.

Wise Yogi Tells Us

Let your children's yoga workout be fun and full of communication when they need it, so they can get the most out of each pose and you'll have a better idea of how they're doing, what they do and don't understand, and how you can best progress with them. When yoga is a family affair, everyone stays in better touch.

Baby Love

Babies are great for cuddling, but they make great *yogis*, too! Babies do some yoga poses all on their own—like the cobra pose, when they look up from a prone position to find the source of a noise. Babies naturally push and test their bodies so they can develop their muscles, mobility, coordination, and dexterity. And you can help your infant optimize this development with some simple yoga moves. Have fun; listen to your baby; and keep the attitude loving, gentle, and responsive.

Put your daughter on her back on a blanket, smile, tell her you are going to do some yoga, then gently take one of her feet in your hand. Wiggle each toe, flex and point her foot, rotate her ankle, flex and straighten her knee, flex and straighten her hip. Move her leg around and around. Pretend her leg is a tree swaying in the breeze (tell her all about it!), or the neck of a loping giraffe, or a slithery snake, or a regal flamingo. Have fun! Then do the same thing on the other leg and each arm. Let your imagination suggest ideas for what your baby's arms and legs could be as you move each limb through its range of motion.

Ouch!

Never force your baby's body in a direction it doesn't want to go. Also pay attention to your baby's response to yoga. If he or she isn't in the mood, try again later.

Turn your baby gently onto her stomach, and using a rattle or your voice, make a noise above her head until she moves her eyes or head, or (if developmentally appropriate) she pushes herself up to see what all the commotion is about. Let her see you or the rattle, and smile.

Babies can even do *shavasana!* Place your son on his back and give him a gentle massage, starting at his feet and working your way around his limbs, then gently rubbing his chest, tummy, and head. Ah, now that's one relaxed baby! (Shh—lights out!)

Toddler Time!

Toddlers are finally able to do yoga poses on their own, although occasionally they will need help from you to figure out how to get into a pose. Toddlers love poses that move, make noise, and help them expend that immense toddler energy. Who knows … you may end up with fewer tantrums on your hands!

Here are a few fun toddler poses to try:

➤ **A Roar, and More!** Everyone get on the hands and knees, sit back on the heels, stick the tongue out as far as possible, and look up. You're all lions, so everybody roar!

➤ **Hop to It!** Everyone squat down on the floor and hop around like frogs. A few "ribbits" offered up to the heavens never hurt anyone.

➤ **Flower Power.** Everyone curl up on the ground like seeds, then imagine being watered and the sun shining. Slowly expand, then rise up out of the ground. Slowly, now! Gradually get taller and taller until head, face, and arms open up into a beautiful bloom.

Peppy Preschoolers

Preschoolers have super-powered imaginations and are developing the coordination, flexibility, and balance to accomplish even more yoga poses. While preschoolers would also enjoy the toddler poses in the preceding section, the following poses are great fun for preschoolers, too, and use preschool skills toddlers haven't quite mastered.

➤ **Mountain's Majesty.** Stand as in the classic mountain pose (Chapter 13). Ask your kids what it feels like to be a mountain. What kind of mountain are they? Rocky and imposing? Rounded, green foothills? Volcano? Is anybody about to explode?

➤ **Be the Tree.** Everyone stand firmly rooted with both feet on the ground (unlike the classic tree pose on one foot). Now let your kids feel how the weather is gradually changing: from sunny and still to windy to blustery to an all-out thunderstorm. How do all the trees shift and move with the weather? Have everyone make appropriate wind and leaf-rustling sounds. Is that a tornado? Woahhhhh! (Don't be surprised if a few trees fall over!)

➤ **Pretty Kitties.** Now be a bunch of cats. Notice how cats move differently than dogs. Lie down. Stretch out. Stand up. Streeeeetch! Try to feel the way a cat feels and move the way a cat moves.

Yoga K–6

Kids in grade school are learning machines, so you can take advantage of those burgeoning minds to really expand the possibilities of a yoga practice. As kids progress through grade school, they become increasingly independent, but you should try to continue practicing with them. A family that practices yoga together is making memories to last a lifetime!

➤ **For the birds.** Each person choose a type of bird, then practice standing, hopping, and flying like that bird. Notice how a sparrow is different from a great blue heron, a mockingbird different from a vulture, a hummingbird different from an eagle. (And remind your kids—birds don't bump into each other!)

➤ **Dog days. Have a dog party!** Everyone chooses a dog, whether poodle or St. Bernard. Run, play, pant, play, roll over, play, and play like the dog you have chosen.

➤ **Invent your own nature poses.** The possibilities are endless.

➤ **Kids can also learn breathing exercises.** But keep it simple. Have kids rest their hands on your stomach to feel how your stomach moves gently when you bring your breath lower. Then have them try this on each other. Ask them if they remember when they were sleeping in the crib and their tummies moved up and down. Ask them to pretend they are in the crib now.

➤ **Kids can even meditate!** Have kids sit quietly and focus on a pleasant object, like a flower, a small figurine, or a toy. At first, rather than stress the absence of thought, suggest that your kids focus on one single feeling, such as love, happiness, or peacefulness. When thoughts arise, refocus on how the feeling *feels* instead.

Ouch!

Kids taking the significant step of starting grade school may be under pressures adults aren't aware of. No longer under our watchful eyes, they can suffer from peer pressure, pressure to succeed, and learning problems—even in kindergarten! Let yoga be a bridge between you and your gradeschooler. It will help your child handle stress and keep the lines of communication open between you.

Teen Yogis

Teenagers can gain great benefit from a regular yoga practice, which will help to keep them physically fit, strong, flexible, and confident. The self-esteem teens can gain from yoga may be the most important benefit of all. Yoga can also help kids develop self-discipline and gain control over their bodies, which are subject to intense hormonal fluctuations and strong emotions during these years.

Teens can do any of the yoga poses adults can do, and often more of them, since teens still have a degree of flexibility adults have allowed to slip away. Encourage your teens to read this book and work through it—with you, on their own, or both. Let yoga be a connection between you and an avenue for communication. Even if they don't always show it, your teens want to connect with you and need to maintain that bond as they move toward becoming adults themselves.

Family Yoga

Lots of yoga poses can be adapted to become group poses. Be a mountain range, a forest of trees, a pack of dogs, a circle of cobras, a school of fish, or a field of cows. Be heroes together in hero pose, form a circle of tortoises, or bob like boats on an open sea in boat pose.

Some yoga poses can be linked. Sit in a meditation circle holding hands, go foot-to-foot in boat pose, head-to-head in fish pose, or rest heads on each other's stomachs in *shavasana*. Combine poses like the downward facing dog over the plank pose, balance the tree pose by standing back-to-back with the mountain pose, or do *vinyasa* like the sun salutation in unison. The possibilities are endless! Flip through this book for ideas, and have a great time.

And at the end of your family yoga session, a group hug!

Ouch!

If you start to hear whines and complaints or sense any reluctance, boredom, or frustration in your kids during your yoga practice, either adjust activities immediately or stop. You don't want to make yoga a negative experience for kids. Fun yoga now could mean a lifetime love of yoga. Yoga that is boring or authoritarian may turn kids off for good. Never push a child into a pose. To kids, poses are play. You might want to try this with your own yoga practice, too! Have fun!

The Least You Need to Know

➤ Men can be great *yogis*—why not take a class?

➤ Yoga can help overcome feelings of aggression, competition, or general dis-satisfaction by offering a satisfying and whole-self physical and spiritual path.

➤ Kids—from infants to teens—can do yoga and learn to love it for a lifetime.

➤ Practice yoga as a family to build memories that will last a lifetime.

Chapter 26

Yoga for Seniors

Maybe you've flipped doubtfully through the pages of this book and have uneasily come to rest on this chapter. You think—you suspect that—you're just too old to do yoga. Isn't yoga for all those limber, energetic young people? Certainly not! Yoga is for everyone, and a regular yoga practice can be of immense physical, mental, emotional, and spiritual benefit to anyone who is experiencing some of the signs of aging (and that's most of us!). Many Indian *yogis* practice well into their hundreds. If yoga can help you live a longer, healthier life, then what have you got to lose?

Even if you've never sat on the floor or meditated, let alone tried the lotus position or the plough or the headstand, you can still give it a try. Let yoga work its magic on your body, your mind, and your spirit.

Yoldies but Goodies!

Senior *yogis* are often the wisest *yogis* of all, even if they're new to yoga. When you've walked the earth for a while, you understand a little more about yourself and about life, suffering, and joy, simply because you've seen more of it. If you haven't practiced yoga before, now is a wonderful time to start.

Aging brings about some undeniable physical changes. As we age, we all lose muscle tissue and bone mass if we don't stay physically active and combat these changes with weight-bearing activities to build muscle and bone. Studies show that bone loss can be reversed through weight-bearing activities like walking (great for hip, leg, knee, ankle, and foot bones and joints); light weight lifting; and of course, yoga poses in which you hold, shift, and manipulate your own body weight.

Practicing yoga can help you protect against bone and muscle loss, prevent the compression fractures common with osteoporosis, and encourage good posture as you age.

Internally, you are experiencing changes, too. The great thing about yoga is that it can balance many of these internal changes in ways you might not even expect. Yoga can smooth digestion that becomes less reliable by stimulating and activating the stomach, colon, abdomen, and internal organs. Your blood vessels lose elasticity, but yoga vinyasa and pranayama techniques suffuse your body with oxygen and increase circulation to keep your entire circulatory system limber. As you age, you may find you don't sleep as well or eat as willingly. A regular yoga practice can make sleep sounder and more rejuvenating, and it can help you work up a healthy appetite, too. Yoga helps bolster a suppressed immune system and keeps all your internal organs stimulated and balanced.

Before beginning your yoga practice (or any exercise program), consult your primary care physician, who will want to follow your progress and coordinate care with your yoga instructor. Many great yoga classes are available now for seniors, which means that poses are adapted and designed to help with the specific concerns and needs of mature *yogis*. Ask at your local YMCA, holistic health center, health club, or senior center. You'll be surprised at how many seniors are already doing yoga!

One of the biggest concerns of people as they age is memory loss. The fear of Alzheimer's disease is widespread, and even simple forgetfulness (where did you put those car keys?) can strike fear into the heart of anybody over 40. As you age, you may have more trouble concentrating and remembering, but much of this is due to stress or the result of simple neglect. When it comes to your brain, it's "use it or lose it." Yoga offers some great ways to use that brain. Balance poses and meditation in particular keep the mind focused, clear, and as limber as a pair of legs folded into the lotus pose.

A Yoga Minute

Deficiencies of vitamins B_6, B_{12}, and folic acid can aggravate or even imitate symptoms of memory loss, Alzheimer's disease, and other forms of senile dementia. Get enough of all three through vitamin supplements and/or food sources such as spinach, broccoli, Brussels sprouts, bananas, carrots, liver, salmon, leafy greens, asparagus, oranges, orange juice, and fortified breakfast cereals. The herb ginkgo biloba has also been shown to improve blood flow to the brain and could combat age-associated memory loss. Ask your doctor about it.

Meditation Power

Seniors are perfect candidates for meditation. Your brain is so full of experiences, information, memories, and ideas that it can really use a break. For a few minutes each day, take some time to yourself to reflect on something beautiful, then let this beautiful reflection gently melt into the breath until breath and peace are all that remain.

Meditation has a wonderfully rejuvenating effect on both your mind and your body. A regular meditation practice will help you think more quickly and clearly, access information more easily, and even enjoy your mental processes more. Your thoughts will come more easily, your memory will be sharper, and you'll find that you handle life with a calm clarity you may never have experienced before.

Proper posture in sitting meditation makes meditation more comfortable and the body less distracting. The easy pose is a simple, basic sitting meditation pose perfect for yoga meditation. Your knees may not come all the way to the ground as Joan is demonstrating, and that's A-OK! Keep the focus on a tall spine. Placing a pillow under your tailbone will help you sit more comfortably, too.

All it takes is a few minutes each day in *shavasana* or sitting meditation. Relax and listen to your breathing. Become aware of the room around you and the body that houses your soul. Don't try to think or feel anything, but if you do, acknowledge it, then let it go. Practice letting your mind relax into a tranquil state, unplagued by worry, anxiety, sadness, or even happiness. Just "be" for a few minutes each day. Life will come into focus, and you'll discover all kinds of things about yourself (and you thought you knew yourself by now!). For more on meditation, see *The Complete Idiot's Guide to Meditation,* also by the authors of this book.

If you are uncomfortable lying flat on the floor due to lower back or joint pain, place a pillow or rolled blanket under your knees and another under your head and neck for support when practicing yoga's shavasana pose.

Yoga Poses for Your Whole Self

Meditation may be all well and good, but maybe you want to get moving first. Great! Any poses you enjoy will be good for your soul, but consider including poses that build bone strength, muscle strength, flexibility, balance, and concentration to keep your muscles, bones, and mind strong.

While we certainly don't assume that just because you are over 65, you are less able to do any pose in this book than someone who is 25, we have adapted some of the following poses to meet the needs of seniors who are new to yoga; may have been living a sedentary life; or suffer from bone loss, muscle weakness, or joint pain. Feel free to take the following suggestions—or not—according to your individual needs.

The following poses are excellent additions to any yoga routine but can be particularly beneficial for seniors (check with your doctor before starting any new exercise program):

➤ **Standing poses are great for developing strength and physical control (see Chapter 13, "What Do You Stand For?").** Try the mountain pose, the three warrior poses, and the lightning bolt pose to start.

➤ **Balance poses (Chapter 13) are excellent for building strength and, once you've mastered them, confidence.** They hone concentration, giving your brain a workout right along with your bones and muscles. The tree pose is a good balance pose to start with. Be patient with yourself. Balance poses will become easier with practice. Don't worry about holding any pose for a long time. Use a wall or chair for support at first if it helps you, then move a few inches away once you feel secure. You can practice other poses while sitting in a chair. Use your imagination, and do what your body tells you it can do.

➤ **Practice the downward facing dog (see Chapter 18, "Take the Forward Path") each day.** It builds upper and lower body strength, and it also has many of the advantages of the inversions. Keep your knees bent. Increase

Ouch!

If you have a serious medical condition, begin your yoga practice with care. Inform both your primary care physician *and* your yoga instructor, so that your yoga practice can be personalized to take your medical needs into full account. In this way, your yoga practice will be more likely to help and not to hinder your path toward healing and well-being.

A Yoga Minute

Balance poses require such minute and complex coordination of so many different muscles and nerves that these poses are as much a workout for the brain as the body. So keep that brain in shape! Crossword puzzles and new learning experiences are great, but add a few balance poses to your daily brain workout, too!

the time in the pose by increasing your breaths. For example, "This week I'll hold the pose for two deep breaths. Next week (or month) I'll take three deep breaths in the pose."

➤ **If your legs tend to be weak, try standing in front of a sturdy chair (preferably one without arms) and practicing the lightning bolt pose (Chapter 13).** Each time you try the lightning bolt variation, come down just a little bit lower. If your legs start to feel weak or shaky, sit down in the chair and take a smile break. Stand up and try again. Slowly develop your thigh and ankle strength this way. If you have trouble reaching your arms over your head, place your hands in *namaste* (prayer) position.

A variation of the lightning bolt pose to strengthen your thighs and ankles.

➤ **You might also find inversions strengthening and empowering.** Once you feel steady and strong in the mountain pose (Chapter 13), move to the bridge, then the shoulderstand, then the plough, and then the headstand (all in Chapter 15, "Come on, Body, Let's Do the Twist"). The headstand isn't as hard as you might think, once you are centered and strong. Don't try it before you feel ready, but once you've done it, do it as often as you can. It will help you feel rejuvenated. Get your doctor's okay on this. Once he or she sees how strong yoga practice is making you, your doctor may want a few yoga lessons!

➤ **When appropriate or necessary, practice sitting poses in a chair for support, but make sure you maintain good posture!** If your back muscles aren't used to working, it may feel better to slump, but bad posture is ultimately more taxing and detrimental to your physical health than good posture. Imagine a string pulling you upward from the crown of your head. Feel as if you are suspended from the string, barely touching the seat of the chair. The longer you do this, the easier it gets and the better it feels.

Stop slumping in that easy chair! Practice sitting poses in a straight-backed chair to keep your spine and back muscles healthy and properly in line. Notice how the chest and internal organs of digestion are compressed in a slouch? Sitting up straight offers your organs a chance to work more efficiently. With practice, you'll find that sitting up straight is more comfortable than a couch potato slouch.

➤ **Practice the sun salutation (Chapter 16, "A Continuous Flow") each morning, and reflect on the sun's power and beauty.** Other *vinyasa* are great for keeping muscles limber and joints mobile, but if any movement or pose is painful, don't continue with it. Arthritis responds well to exercise, but particularly inflamed joints shouldn't be aggravated.

➤ **Water yoga is lots of fun and helps protect bones, muscles, and joints from jarring or taking on too much weight.** Many yoga poses can be adapted for different depths of water. Try standing poses in chest-deep water, sitting poses in shallow water (see the following figures). Let the water help you with the poses, and let the water's movement soothe and relax you. Your yoga teacher might even be willing to hold an occasional class at the pool or the beach. It never hurts to ask!

➤ **Who says walking can't be yoga?** Walk with intention, focus, concentration, and mindfulness, and your daily walk in the fresh air can become a meditation session and a lesson in life. So much to see, hear, smell, feel, so much beauty, so much activity or quiet, so many or so few people or animals. Let your surroundings speak to you, teach you, communicate with you. Walk through the world awake, with your mind and your eyes wide open. Talk about a great workout!

➤ **The child's pose is incredibly relaxing, but it may be hard on your knees.** Try the child's pose on two chairs with folded blankets or pillows for cushioning (see the following figure). Why shouldn't you do the child's pose? You *are* young at heart!

311

Joan assists a friend in a supported water yoga spinal twist.

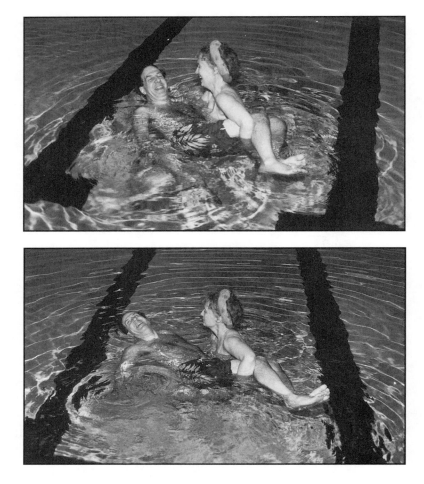

This refreshing supported child's pose stretch gives instant relief!

➤ **Lie still in *shavasana* (see Chapter 19, "Dead to the World") every day for at least 10 minutes.** This pose teaches your body and your mind how to release their tensions and troubles, simplifying your existence and moving toward unity. Everything will work better after a little *shavasana!*

Overall, keep in mind your particular areas of strength and weakness, then tailor your yoga program to balance both. Having lived on the earth for an impressive number of years should not keep you from attempting yoga. In fact, many *yogis* live to be over 100 years old and still practice each day. Don't forget breathing exercises and meditation, as well as reflections on the *yamas* and *niyamas* (see Chapter 6, "Walking Yoga's Eightfold Path"). Practice outside whenever you can, and pay attention to the natural world around you. Your fitness program, as well as your life, will be whole, balanced, peaceful, and filled with bliss.

Having the Time of Your Life

Whether you are 40 or 60 or 80 or 100, age is just a number. You know that old cliché about being only as young as you feel? How true it is (maybe that's why it became a cliché!). Even a 20-year-old can feel old if he never exercises, never breathes deeply, doesn't eat right, and doesn't live mindfully.

Wise Yogi Tells Us

The National Council on the Aging and the International Longevity Center conducted a survey of 3,000 adults in the United States, called *Myths and Realities of Aging 2000.* The survey found that most Americans would be happy if they lived to be 90, and 44 percent of respondents described the present as the best years of their lives—a 32 percent increase over results from the 1974 survey. The survey also revealed that most Americans favor spending more money rather than less on older people; that older people are less worried about their health, finances, and the threat of crime than they were 25 years ago; and that in the minds of many, old age begins with declining physical or mental ability, not with the arrival of a specific age.

Much of what we become is a matter of habit. We get out of the habit of exercising, or eating right, or paying attention, and slowly it becomes part of our lives. The great thing is that it works the other way, too. The more we get in the habit of moving;

eating well; paying attention; and living with purpose, compassion, and spirit, the better our lives will become.

So you say you are too old to be this or that? So what? The world is full of possibilities, opportunities, and joy. If you can't do one thing, do something else. Everyone, at any age, is limited by certain factors in life. Don't let your limits stop you. Let your abilities get you started and keep you going. Open your breath, lengthen your spine, open your chest, expand your mind.

Coping with Loss and Grief

Eventually, we all have to deal with loss and grief. The longer we're here on this planet, the more we will need to learn how to handle loss: the loss of loved ones, or health, or independence. These are all very real issues each one of us will need to confront at some time, whether for ourselves or to help another.

Yoga helps us simplify our lives, our emotions, and our material concerns. The study of yoga can help us gain perspective on what is important. It can help us detach from our competitive selves and see our bodies and minds as oases of self-discovery. *Shavasana*, the corpse pose (Chapter 19), helps us to explore death within life. We can also discover that the limits of our body do not define our existence. Our existence is interconnected with the joys and sorrows of all life, including the bee on the porch, the bird in the air, the snake on the path, the fish in the water. Letting ourselves be with, and be one with, all of life can open up truth to our minds and hearts. We may not know you personally, but we know one thing about you: You are worth the effort required to make a regular life into a great life. It's never too late to start living; to start practicing yoga; to start moving and bending and stretching and lifting; to start focusing, concentrating, breathing deeply, and meditating. And that's just the beginning of your transformation. There's no telling what you can accomplish with a body, mind, and spirit in full throttle.

We aren't saying you should take up skydiving or bungee jumping or water skiing (unless you really want to). But we are saying that your life is what you make it, and those who think they can't make much of their lives aren't using their imaginations. Anyone can find meaning, fulfillment, and joy in life. But you won't find it if you don't look for it. The first part of every yoga pose is visualization, and it's amazing where that visualization can lead.

So let yoga help you look. Let yoga bless you with daily renewal, energy, tranquility, contentment, even bliss. Let yoga help you to find the real you, which is ageless, timeless, and complete. That "you" can do anything. We know it. And we wouldn't want to stand in your way!

The Least You Need to Know

➤ Yoga is an excellent way of life for seniors, improving physical, mental, emotional, and spiritual well-being.

➤ Meditation can bring clarity of mind to seniors, improving memory and making information seem more accessible.

➤ Yoga poses that increase muscle and bone strength, flexibility, balance, and concentration are excellent for seniors.

➤ Yoga can help anyone cope with loss and grief, as it encourages a move toward a simpler, more unified existence.

➤ This can be the best time of your life!

Schedule

8-11 Work
11-11:05 Coffee
11:06-1 More work
1-1:15 Lunch
1:16-8 Work
8-11 House work
11-12 Yoga
12-5 Sleep
5 Get up, repeat.

Yoga Sessions for the Time You Have

Here are some great ideas for routines to begin your yoga practice, based on the yoga classes that Joan teaches to her students. Whether you need a relaxing five-minute break in the middle of the workday, or an invigorating full-hour session at home to get you energized, toned, and ready for anything, Joan has suggestions for you. Each sequence of yoga postures helps you focus on something specific. For example, one sequence can hone in on improving your physical sense of balance, while another can help you release anger and negative feelings. Other examples include toning internal organs, building upper body strength, and increasing lung capacity. You'll want to choose the routine that's right for you. And remember, it's not important *how much* yoga you do, but that you keep practicing, doing as much as you can whenever you can. Yoga moves at *your* pace, in the time *you* have!

Every Day Is a New Opportunity to Grow

Every time you practice yoga, try to view it as the *first* time. Study what your body is doing, and don't take anything for granted. Yoga is a new experience every day! Let's say you've learned the mountain pose, *tadasana,* but you think it's an easy pose and you don't concentrate on it very much during your practice. Your performance of the pose becomes unaware, and your yoga practice is likely to be unproductive. Every time you enter this mountain pose, enter it fully. Feel your thigh muscles strong and engaged, reach through your fingertips toward the ground where each toe is securely planted, lower your shoulders, and feel your head and neck rise upward; you are a mountain!

Also put aside any preconceived ideas you have about being a "beginning student," "intermediate student," or "advanced student." Sure, some postures might be beyond your reach right now, but yoga is a *personal* journey. The length of time you hold poses in comfort—whatever their degree of complexity—and how grounded you are in the poses are the closest things to "advancement" in performing *Hatha Yoga*. The evenness and strength of your breath are also reflections of the depth of your study. Approach your body as a new and special friend with every yoga class. Be sensitive and kind to yourself, and your yoga practice is sure to prosper.

Let's get started!

Five-Minute Yoga Sessions

These sessions are good at home or at work—any time you need a quick lift or a refocusing boost to help find your center!

Session 1

Try five minutes of breathwork doing alternate nostril breathing. The time will fly by, and you will begin to feel quietly balanced (*Hatha*).

Session 2

Stand in the mountain pose and bend over into the triangle pose. Hold the triangle on the right side for five breaths, then do the left side for five breaths. Go back into the mountain pose and study your alignment.

Session 3

Face a wall, and reach your arms out to place your palms on the wall at shoulder height. Take a big step back, and bend at the hips toward the wall. Lengthen your spine. This is the downward facing dog against the wall! Hold this position for five minutes. This is a great way to energize your body and open those stiff shoulders.

15-Minute Yoga Sessions

The 15-minute practice is great when you're in a rush and don't have too much time to spare. It may be hard at first to find the time, but we bet you'll end up cherishing this quarter-hour as your indispensable yoga haven! Hold every pose for at least five breaths. Try flowing into each consecutive posture.

Session 1

This sequence builds strength and is a quick way of releasing anger that has turned inward. Use it to help purge negative feelings.

➤ Mountain pose

➤ Warrior 1 pose (both sides)

➤ Warrior 2 pose (both sides)

➤ Side angle stretch (both sides)

➤ Mountain pose

Session 2

This sequence is good for relaxing, calming, and quieting down. It tones the internal organs of the chest and abdomen.

➤ Lying down spinal twist

➤ Leg lifts

➤ *Shavasana*

Session 3

This session focuses on meditation and internal reflection.

➤ *Yoga mudra*

➤ Camel pose

➤ Meditative pose (Pick the one you feel most comfortable in.)

Session 4

This session uses *pranayama* techniques to open your heart *chakra,* deepening your feelings of love and opening your chest with the breath.

➤ Alternate nostril breathing

➤ *Om* exhalation

➤ *Shavasana*

30-Minute Yoga Sessions

Build up to 30-minute sessions at least one or two times per week. Try to hold each pose for six full breaths. If you can, reserve a regular time and place for these nurturing yoga sessions. You deserve it!

Session 1

This session is an upper body workout performed mostly on the floor, opening your chest and heart with the downward facing dog pose to balance the sequence.

➤ *Shavasana.*

➤ Bridge.

➤ Plough.

➤ Fish.

➤ Child's pose.

➤ Repeat this sequence twice, for a total of three rounds.

➤ Cobra.

➤ Child's pose.

➤ Downward facing dog.

➤ Child's pose.

➤ Repeat this sequence twice, for a total of three rounds.

➤ *Shavasana.*

Session 2

Energize and strengthen your body with this invigorating session.

1. Child's pose.
2. Single leg lifts.
3. Double leg lifts.
4. Lying down spinal twist.
5. Bring your knees to your chest, hold there, and pause.
6. Turn over and go into the cobra three times, each time holding the pose a bit longer.
7. Move into the downward facing dog.
8. Step one foot forward, straighten your legs, turn to the side, and come up into a triangle.
9. Do the triangle on both sides.
10. Move into the lightening bolt.
11. Come back down into the child's pose.
12. Repeat the entire sequence of poses two times, for a total of three rounds.
13. Rest in *shavasana.*

Session 3

This session concentrates on the Jupiter *chakra* and helps balance sexual energy.

➤ *Yoga mudra*
➤ Hero
➤ Mountain
➤ Triangle
➤ Eagle
➤ Cow
➤ *Yoga mudra*
➤ *Shavasana*

Session 4

The Mars *chakra*—the *chakra* of action located at the center of the body—is stimulated in this session, catapulting the body to energy!

➤ Three slow full rounds of sun salutations
➤ Camel
➤ Boat
➤ *Shavasana*

Session 5

The Mercury *chakra*—the *chakra* of communication located at the throat—is activated in this session to help improve interactions with others.

➤ Half spinal twist
➤ Shoulderstand
➤ Plough
➤ Bridge
➤ *Shavasana*

Full-Hour Yoga Sessions

Congratulations! You're about to luxuriate in a full hour of yoga practice. We bet you'll find that this one hour devoted to centering, strengthening, and fostering the yoga mind/body connection will make the other hours in your day far more productive and fulfilling!

321

Session 1

1. Stand tall in the mountain pose, toes spread, knees lifted, and shoulders relaxed down. Do head and shoulder rolls.

2. Like a rag doll, reach your hands to the ceiling and let them fall to the floor; keep your muscles loose and don't worry about touching your toes. Rag doll helps you warm up, increasing alertness by bringing blood to the brain and overcoming stiffness in the spine and legs. Return to the mountain pose to regain focus.

3. Jump your feet about a yard apart for the triangle pose. Perform the triangle on both sides. Return to the mountain pose.

4. From the mountain pose, bend your right knee out, and place your right foot on your left thigh to move into the tree pose. Bring your palms together in front of your heart, and then raise them over your head while retaining your balance. Return to the mountain pose.

5. Walk to a wall in the room and place your hands on the wall at shoulder height. Take a giant step backward. Slowly bend at the waist, keeping the natural alignment of the spine to lengthen into the downward facing dog against the wall. Return to the mountain pose.

6. Turn around to face away from the wall. Jump your feet apart about a yard. Place your hands on your hips, and bend forward slowly with a flat back. The legs stay active, and the back retains its natural alignment. You are a tabletop! Move into the downward facing dog and hold for five breaths.

7. Move into the child's pose. Rise into the downward facing dog. Repeat three times, holding the downward facing dog for a longer period in each repetition.

8. Rest in *shavasana.*

Session 2

1. Begin in *shavasana.* Concentrate on breathing from the diaphragm. Let go of all thoughts, and relax each part of your body, from your toes to your head.

2. Prepare for leg lifts by lifting one knee to your chest, hugging it, and raising your head toward the knee. Hold for three seconds. Repeat with the other leg. This pose is called *pavana maktasana* in Sanskrit; it is a wind-relieving pose, which massages the intestines. Now perform single and double leg lifts.

3. Move into the hero pose and follow with the cow pose. Hero benefits the knees and tones the thighs. Cow stimulates the nerves at the base of the spine, preventing calcifying and aging. Cow also stimulates the nerves in the feet.

4. Now move into the butterfly pose to stretch the inner hips and thighs—a revitalizing pose.

5. Stand erect in the mountain pose.

6. Jump your feet three to four feet apart for warrior 2. Perform on both sides.

7. Return to the mountain pose.

8. Jump your feet out again, this time for warrior 1. Reach toward the heavens, but stay grounded on earth.

9. Return to the mountain pose.

10. Move into the standing head to knees pose, a forward bend. Hold for as long as you can comfortably.

11. Rest in *shavasana*.

Glossary

This glossary is divided into two sections to help you find the terms you need quickly and efficiently. The first section includes all of the Sanskrit yoga terms you've learned in *The Complete Idiot's Guide to Yoga, Second Edition.* The second section includes more terms related to yoga and health that you'll want to remember. Use both sections of the glossary as quick reference tools and easy ways to look up whatever you need to know.

Sanskrit Terms

abhinivesha   Survival instinct.

adho mukha shvanasana   Downward facing dog; a forward bend.

adho mukha vrksasana   The handstand; an inversion.

ahimsa   One of the *yamas;* nonviolence.

ananda-maya-kosha   The bliss sheath and fifth sheath of existence.

anna-maya-kosha   The physical body and first sheath of existence.

apana   A type of *prana;* the vital energy of excretion that flows downward and out of the body, ridding it of impurities.

aparigraha   One of the *yamas;* nongreed.

ardha baddha padma pashchimottanasana   Bound half lotus pose; a seated forward bending pose.

ardha baddha padmottanasana   Standing half bound lotus pose; an advanced balancing pose.

asanas   The postures, or exercises, of yoga designed to help you master control of your body.

Ashtanga Yoga   Literally refers to the Eight Limbs of Yoga; in Western culture, this type of yoga has come to mean a *Hatha Yoga* practice that includes an intense *vinyasa* workout.

asmita   Ego or individuality.

asteya   One of the *yamas;* nonstealing.

avidya   Incorrect comprehension.

baddha konasana   The butterfly; a sitting posture.

baddha padmasana   The bound lotus; a meditative pose.

bandha   Literally "to bind" or "to lock," *bandhas* are muscular locks used during postures and breathing exercises to intensify the energy of *prana* so it can eliminate impurities from the body.

Bhagavad Gita   One of India's most beloved and famous sacred texts, this is the epic story of Arjuna, a warrior-prince who confronts moral dilemmas and is led to a better understanding of reality through the intercession of the god *Krishna*.

Bhakti Yoga   Sincere, heartfelt devotion to the divine is the primary focus of this type of yoga.

bhastrika   Literally "bellows," *bhastrika* is a breathing technique that imitates the action of a bellows.

bhramari   Also known as *bee breath,* this breathing technique imitates the sound of a bee.

bhujangasana   The cobra; a backbend.

brahmacharya   One of the *yamas;* chastity or nonlust.

brahman   The absolute, or divinity itself.

buddhi   The intellect.

chakras   Centers of energy that exist between the base of your spinal column and the crown of your head.

cakrasana   The wheel; a backbend.

chandra namaskara   Moon salutation; a *vinyasa*.

dandasana   The staff; a sitting posture.

dhanurasana   The bow; a backbend.

dharana   Orienting the mind toward a single point.

dhyana Meditation, or the process of quieting the mind to free yourself from pre-conceptions and illusions.

duhkha Pain, suffering, trouble, and discomfort; a mental state during which limitations and a profound sense of dissatisfaction are perceived.

dvesha Refusal.

garudasana The eagle; a balance posture.

ghee Clarified butter, or butter from which all solids have been removed, leaving only the oil; a traditional Indian food.

gomukhasana The cow; a sitting posture.

gunas The three primary qualities existing in the universe—*sattva, rajas,* and *tamas*—can apply to the mind and to influences on the body, such as food.

guru Literally "dispeller of darkness," a *guru* is a personal spiritual advisor who helps direct the *yogi* toward enlightenment.

halasana The plough; an inversion.

Hatha Yoga A type of yoga primarily concerned with mastering control over the physical body as a path to enlightenment; *Hatha Yoga* combines opposing forces to achieve balance.

Hatha-Yoga-Pradipika A fourteenth-century, comprehensive guide to *Hatha Yoga*.

ida A channel on the left side of the spine through which *prana* moves.

ishvara-pranidhana One of the *niyamas;* centering on the divine.

jalandhara bandha A *bandha* that locks the throat.

janu shirshasana Sitting one leg; a forward bend.

japa The process of repeating a *mantra* over and over for the purpose of clearing the mind.

Jnana Yoga This type of yoga emphasizes questioning, meditation, and contemplation as paths to enlightenment.

Jupiter chakra Located on the spine near the genitals, this energy center involves water, sexuality, passion, the creation of life, and taste.

kali yuga The fourth of four ages (*yuga* means "age"), and the age in which we are now living; the shortest of all the ages, *kali yuga* is 432,000 years long.

kapalabhati A cleansing ritual for the respiratory tract, lungs, and sinuses; also called *skull shining.*

karma The law of cause and effect, or the movement toward balanced consciousness; everything you do, say, or even think has an immediate effect on the universe that will reverberate back to you in some way.

Karma Yoga Selfless action and service to others are emphasized in this type of yoga.

Kevali Kumbhaka A *pranayama* technique involving retaining the breath, it helps increase breath control and lung capacity.

koshas The five sheaths of existence that comprise the body.

Krishna A popular Hindu god.

Kriya Yoga The yoga of action and participation in life.

kundalini Literally "she who is coiled," *kundalini* is a psychospiritual energy force in the body that is often compared to a snake lying curled at the base of the spine, waiting to be awakened. When fully awakened, it is said to actually restructure the body, allowing the *yogi* to control previously involuntary bodily functions.

Kundalini Yoga This esoteric and mystical form of yoga is centered around awakening and employing *kundalini* energy.

kurmasana The tortoise; a forward bend.

mandalas Beautiful, usually circular, geometric designs that draw your eye to the center and are used as a center of focus in meditation.

mano-maya-kosha The mind sheath and third sheath of existence.

mantra A sound or sounds that resonate in the body and evoke certain energies during meditation.

Mantra Yoga The chanting of *mantras* characterizes this type of yoga.

maricyasana The half spinal twist; a twisting pose.

Mars chakra Located on the spine behind the navel, this energy center is associated with digestion or "gastric fire," your sense of self, and physical actions.

matsyasana The fish; a backbend.

Matsyendra A Hindu sage and one of the first teachers of *Hatha Yoga*.

Mercury chakra Located in the throat, this energy center governs communication.

moon chakra Located behind your head at the base of your skull, the moon *chakra* complements the sun *chakra*. Energy enters the moon *chakra*, travels down to the Saturn *chakra*, then rises up and exits the sun *chakra*.

mudhasana Child's pose; a forward bend.

mudras Hand gestures that direct the life current through the body.

mula bandha An anal lock.

murccha kumbkhaka A *pranayama* technique also known as third eye breathing, this exercise involves breathing with a focus on the third eye, or the area between and just above the eyebrows (the sixth *chakra*).

nadi shodhana   A breathing exercise in which nostrils are alternated for inhalation and exhalation.

nadis   Subtle vibratory passages of psychospiritual energy.

namaste mudra   A *mudra* in which the hands are placed together in prayer-like fashion to honor the inner light.

naukasana   The full boat; a balance pose.

nauli   A cleansing ritual for the inner abdomen.

niyamas   Five observances or personal disciplines, as defined by Patanjali in his *Yoga Sutras;* the *niyamas* are *shauca, santosha, tapas, svadhyaya,* and *ishvar-pranidhana.*

Om   A sacred syllable commonly used as a *mantra* during meditation and representative of the absolute or oneness of the universe; a rough approximation of the sound of the universe's vibration.

padma shirshasana   The lotus headstand; an inversion.

padmasana   The lotus pose, a meditative posture in which the legs are crossed and each foot is placed on the opposite thigh; the pose is said to resemble the perfection of the lotus flower.

parshvottanasana   The side angle stretch; a standing posture.

pavana maktasana   Also called wind relieving pose, this standing pose brings the knee to the chest, with head extended toward the knee.

pingala   A channel on the right side of the spine through which *prana* moves.

prana   A form of energy in the universe that animates all physical matter, including the human body; the vital energy of respiration and the soul of the universe.

prana-maya-kosha   The vital body and second sheath of existence.

pranayama   Breathing exercises designed to help you master control of your breath.

pratyahara   Withdrawal of the senses.

purvottanasana   The hands to feet pose; a variation of the plough; an inversion.

raga   Attachment.

Raja Yoga   Also known as The Royal Path, this type of yoga emphasizes control of the intellect to attain enlightenment.

rajas   The quality of high activity and agitation; a *guna.*

Rig-Veda   Literally "Knowledge of Praise," the *Rig-Veda* consists of 1,028 hymns and is the oldest known reference to yoga, and possibly the oldest known text in the world.

roga   Sickness.

samadhi   The state of meditation in which ego disappears and all becomes one; a state of absolute bliss.

samyama   When in a state of *samyama,* the *yogi* has investigated, concentrated on, meditated upon, and contemplated an object or subject until everything about it is known and understood.

santosha   One of the *niyamas;* contentment.

sarvangasana   The shoulderstand; an inversion.

sattva   The quality of clarity and lightness; a *guna.*

Saturn chakra   Located just above the anus at the base of the spine, this energy center involves elimination and your sense of smell.

satya   One of the *yamas;* truthfulness.

setu bandha sarvangasana   The bridge; an inversion.

shat kriyas   Purification rituals.

shauca   One of the *niyamas;* purity, or inner and outer cleanliness.

shavasana   Also known as the *corpse pose,* this pose is meant to bring the body and mind into total, conscious relaxation.

shirshasana   The headstand; an inversion.

shodhana   *Yogic* cleansing rituals.

sitali   A breathing technique involving rolling the tongue, then inhaling through it like a straw; a cooling technique.

sitar   A stringed instrument from India, similar to a mandolin.

sthala basti   A yoga cleansing ritual for the colon, also called ground colon cleansing, involving the churning of the abdominal muscles.

sthira   Steadiness and alertness.

sukha   Lightness and comfort.

sukhasana   Easy pose; a meditative pose.

Sun chakra   Located in the middle of your brow, this energy center is also known as the *third eye,* or center of unclouded perception.

surya namaskara   Sun salutation; a *vinyasa.*

sushumna   A hollow passageway between *pingala* and *ida* that runs through the spinal cord, and through which *kundalini* can travel once it is awakened.

svadhyaya   One of the *niyamas;* the process of inquiring into your own nature, the nature of your beliefs, and the nature of the world's spiritual journey.

svamin   A title of respect for a spiritual person who is master of her- or himself rather than others.

svasthya   Health.

swami   The Anglicized form of *svamin*.

Swami Vivekananda   A *guru* from India who addressed the Parliament of Religions in 1893, and quickly became a popular figure; he was followed by a number of other *swamis* who came to the United States to teach and guide Westerners along the Eastern path of yoga.

tadasana   The mountain; a standing posture.

tamas   The quality of heaviness and inactivity; a *guna*.

Tantra Yoga   This type of yoga is characterized by certain rituals designed to awaken the *kundalini*.

tapas   One of the *niyamas;* self-discipline.

thousand petaled lotus chakra   Located at the crown of the skull, this energy center is the core of self-realization, perspective, unity, and enlightenment.

Transcendental Meditation   Also known as TM, this form of meditation involves the mental repetition of a *mantra*.

trikonasana   The triangle or happy pose; a standing posture.

uddiyana bandha   A *bandha* that locks the abdomen.

ujjayi   A breathing exercise that produces sound in the throat with the inhalation; literally, "she who is victorious."

Upanishads   Scriptures of ancient Hindu philosophy.

urdhvamukha shvanasana   The upward facing dog; a backbend

ustrasana   The camel; a backbend.

utkatasana   The lightning bolt; a standing posture.

uttanasana   Standing head to knee; a forward bend.

uttanatavasana   Leg lifts.

vajrasana   Kneeling pose; a meditative pose.

vashisthasana   The arm balance; a balance posture.

Venus chakra   Located behind your heart, this energy center is the seat of your compassion.

vidya   Correct understanding.

vijnana-maya-kosha   The intellect sheath and fourth sheath of existence.

vinyasa   A steady flow of connected yoga *asanas* linked with breathwork in a continuous movement; a particularly dynamic form of yoga.

virabhadrasana   The warrior; a standing posture.

virasana   The hero; a sitting posture.

vrikshasana   The tree; a balance posture.

vyadhi   Disease.

yamas   Five abstinences that purify the body and mind, as defined by Patanjali in his *Yoga Sutras;* the *yamas* are *ahimsa, satya, asteya, brahmacharya,* and *aparigraha.*

yoga mudra   A forward bend.

Yoga Sutras of Patanjali   The source of Patanjali's Eightfold Path, this collection of succinct aphorisms has largely defined the modern concept of yoga.

yogi   Someone who practices yoga.

yogic   An adjective describing things that are associated with yoga.

yogini   A female *yogi.*

More Terms You'll Want to Know

adrenal glands   A pair of glands located just above the kidneys (in mammals); these glands secrete epinephrine (a stimulant) and certain steroids.

afferent nerves   The nerves that carry messages from the body to the brain.

allopathic medicine   The traditional medicine of Western culture, which focuses on a specific disease or problem and treats it.

Alzheimer's disease   A degenerative brain disease most common in the elderly.

astral body   The vehicle of the spirit, corresponding with the mind; higher than the physical body, but below the causal body.

causal body   The subtlest body, it houses the spirit; higher than the physical and astral bodies.

circadian rhythms   The physiological rhythms people experience throughout the course of a 24-hour day.

deltoids   Muscles that lift and rotate the arms.

diaphragm   A large, flat muscle at the base of the thoracic cavity that controls breathing.

estrogen   Several hormones that produce sexual changes in female mammals.

fruitarian   A person who practices a form of vegetarianism in which no animal products whatsoever are consumed, and all foods must be consumed raw.

holistic medicine   An approach to medicine in which the patient's entire lifestyle, environment, and personality are considered in the treatment of disease.

intercostals   Muscles that expand the ribs.

lacto-ovo-vegetarianism   A form of vegetarianism in which no meat, poultry, or fish is consumed; but eggs, milk, and milk products are consumed.

lacto-vegetarianism   A form of vegetarianism in which no meat, poultry, fish, or eggs are consumed; but milk and milk products are consumed.

larynx   The area of the throat containing the vocal cords.

ligaments   Bands of tissue connecting bones to bones or holding organs in place.

menopause   The period in a woman's life, usually somewhere between the late thirties and the early sixties, when menstruation ceases.

Occident   The West (Europe and the Americas), as opposed to the Orient.

Orient   The East (Asia), as opposed to the Occident.

patella   The kneecap.

pectorals   Chest muscles that pull in and rotate the arms.

physical body   The lowest of the three bodies, the physical body is the body we see; the other bodies are the astral body and the causal body.

pituitary gland   A gland attached to the brain that secretes hormones affecting growth.

PMS   An acronym for premenstrual syndrome.

postpartum depression   A condition experienced by at least 50 percent of new mothers; characterized by depression, anxiety, drastic mood swings, and spontaneous weeping in the week after childbirth.

premenstrual syndrome   A syndrome experienced by some women one to two weeks before the onset of menstruation; symptoms may include irritability, depression, restlessness, back pain, bloating, and swelling.

sartorius   The muscle that twists the thigh and bends the hip and knee.

scapula   The shoulder blade.

sciatic nerve   A long nerve that starts in the hip and runs down the leg.

sciatica   A painful condition felt in the hip or thigh and down the back of the leg, resulting from inflammation of the sciatic nerve.

sensory nerves   The nerves that carry messages from the brain to the body.

sprain   An injury to a ligament.

sternum   The breastbone, a flat bone to which the ribs are attached.

strain   An injury to a muscle or its tendon.

tendon   Tough, connective tissue attaching muscles to bones.

thoracic cavity   The cavity containing your lungs and heart.

thyroid gland   Located near the trachea, this gland secretes hormones that affect growth.

tibia   The inner and thicker bone of the two bones of the lower leg.

tibialis anterior   Muscles that raise the foot.

trachea   The passageway through which air travels after inhalation.

ulna   The larger of the two bones of the forearm.

veganism   A form of vegetarianism in which no animal products of any kind are consumed.

vegetarianism   A diet in which no meat is consumed.

Further Along the Yoga Path: Suggested Reading

Welcome! Now that you've begun your yoga practice with *The Complete Idiot's Guide to Yoga, Second Edition,* no doubt you'll want to read more about the many aspects of yoga, find out how to incorporate yoga into your everyday life, and enhance your yoga practice. Here's a great list of books to help guide you on your yoga path!

Balch, James. F. and Phyllis A. Balch. *Prescription for Nutritional Healing, 2nd Edition.* Garden City Park, New York: Avery Publishing Group, Inc., 1996.

Ballentine, Rudolph. *Transition to Vegetarianism.* Honesdale, Pennsylvania: The Himalayan Institute Press, 1999.

Bender Birch, Beryl. *Beyond Power Yoga: 8 Levels of Practice for Body and Soul.* New York: Fireside, 2000.

——. *Power Yoga.* New York: Simon & Schuster, 1995.

Bhagavad Gita (multiple translations available)

Bstan-'dzin-rgya-mtsho, Dalai Lama XIV (His Holiness the Dalai Lama). *The Art of Happiness.* New York: Riverhead Books, 1998.

Bstan-'dzin-rgya-mtsho, Dalai Lama XIV (His Holiness the Dalai Lama). *Healing Anger.* Ithaca, New York: Snow Lion Publications, 1997.

Budilovsky, Joan and Eve Adamson. *The Complete Idiot's Guide to Massage.* Indianapolis, Indiana: Alpha Books, 1998.

——. *The Complete Idiot's Guide to Meditation.* Indianapolis, Indiana: Alpha Books, 1999.

Budilovsky, Joan. *Fat-Free Yoga.* Oak Brook, Illinois: YOYOGA!, 1997.

——. *The Little Yogi Energy Book.* Oak Brook, Illinois: YOYOGA!, 1997.

——. *Yoga for a New Day.* Oak Brook, Illinois: YOYOGA!, 1996.

Carper, Jean. *Jean Carper's Total Nutrition Guide.* New York: Bantam Books, 1987.

Cheaney, Lee Ann. *Visits Caring for an Aging Parent: Reflections and Advice.* New York: Three Rivers Press, 1998.

Chopra, Deepak. *Ageless Body, Timeless Mind.* New York: Harmony Books, 1993.

Choudhury, Bikram. *Bikram's Beginning Yoga Class.* New York: G.P. Putnam's Sons, 1978.

Christensen, Alice. *The Easy Does It Yoga Trainer's Guide.* Sarasota, Florida: American Yoga Association, 1995.

——. *Yoga of the Heart.* New York: Daybreak Books, 1998.

Couch, Jean. *The Runner's Yoga Book.* Berkeley, California: Rodmell Press, 1990.

de Mello, Anthony. *Wellsprings: A Book of Spiritual Exercises.* New York: Doubleday, 1984.

——. *Awareness: The Perils and Opportunities of Reality.* New York: Doubleday, 1992.

——. *Sadhana, A Way to God: Christian Exercises in Eastern Form.* New York: Doubleday, 1984.

Desikachar, T.K.V. *The Heart of Yoga: Developing a Personal Practice.* Rochester, Vermont: Inner Traditions International, 1995.

Duff, Gail. *Eating Vegetarian: A Step by Step Guide.* Great Britain: Element Books Limited, 1999.

Farhi, Donna. *The Breathing Book: Good Health and Vitality Through Essential Breath Work.* New York: Henry Holt and Company, 1996.

Feuerstein, Georg. *The Shambhala Guide to Yoga*. Boston: Shambhala Publications, Inc., 1996.

———. *The Yoga-Sutra of Patanjali, A New Translation and Commentary*. Rochester, Vermont: Inner Traditions, International, 1979.

Flinders, Carol Lee. *At the Root of this Longing: Reconciling a Spiritual Hunger and a Feminist Thirst*. San Francisco: HarperSanFrancisco, 1998.

Gandhi, Mahatma. *All Men Are Brothers*. India: Navajivan Publishing House, 1960.

Gandhi, Mohandask. *Gandhi's Health Guide*. Freedom, California: The Crossing Press.

Gunther, Bernard. *Energy Ecstasy and Your Seven Vital Chakras*. North Hollywood, California: Newcastle Publishing, 1983.

Hanh, Thich Nhat. *Peace is Every Step*. New York: Bantam Books, 1991.

Hanna, Thomas. *Somatics*. Reading, Massachusetts: Addison Wesley, 1988.

Harrar, Sari and Sara Altshul O'Donnell. *The Woman's Book of Healing Herbs*. Emmaus, Pennsylvania: Rodale Press, Inc., 1999.

Harvey, Andrew. *The Essential Mystics: The Soul's Journey into Truth*. San Francisco: HarperSanFrancisco, 1996.

Hewitt, James. *Teach Yourself Yoga*. Lincolnwood (Chicago): NTC Publishing Group, 1993.

Hittleman, Richard. *Yoga for Health: The Total Program*. New York: Ballantine Books, 1983.

Iyengar, B.K.S. *Light on Yoga*. New York: Schocken Books, 1979.

Japananda, Swami K. *Yoga, You, Your New Life*. Chicago: The Temple of Kriya Yoga, 1981.

Kabat-Zinn, Jon, Ph.D. *Full Catastrophe Living: Using the Wisdom of Your Body and Mind to Face Stress, Pain, and Illness*. New York: Delta, 1990.

Komitor, Jodi and Eve Adamson. *The Complete Idiot's Guide to Yoga with Kids*. Indianapolis, Indiana: Alpha Books, 2000.

Kriyanada, Goswami. *Extraordinary Spiritual Potential*. Chicago: The Temple of Kriya Yoga, 1988.

——. *The Laws of Karma*. Chicago: The Temple of Kriya Yoga, 1995.

——. *The Spiritual Science of Kriya Yoga*. Chicago: The Temple of Kriya Yoga, 1992.

Kriyananda, Sri (J. Donald Walters). *Yoga Postures for Higher Awareness*. Nevada City, California: Crystal Clarity, 1967.

Lasater, Judith, Ph.D. *Relax and Renew*. Berkeley, California: Rodmell Press, 1995.

Lerner, Michael. *Choices in Healing: Integrating the Best of Conventional and Complementary Approaches to Cancer*. Cambridge, Massachusetts: MIT Press, 1994.

LeVert, Suzanne and Gary McClain, Ph.D. *The Complete Idiot's Guide to Breaking Bad Habits, Second Edition*. Indianapolis, Indiana: Alpha Books, 2001.

Levitt, Atma JoAnne. *The Kripalu Cookbook*. Stockbridge, Massachusetts: Berkshire House Publishers, 1995.

Living Yoga: A Comprehensive Guide for Daily Life. Edited by Georg Feuerstein and Stephan Bodian with the staff of *Yoga Journal*. New York: Jeremy P. Tarcher/Perigee Books, 1993.

Mahabharata (numerous translations available).

McClain, Gary R., Ph.D., and Eve Adamson. *The Complete Idiot's Guide to Zen Living*. Indianapolis, Indiana: Alpha Books, 2000.

McLaren, Karla. *Rebuilding the Garden*. Columbia, California: Laughing Tree Press, 1997.

Mehta, Silva and Shyam Mihra. *Yoga the Iyengar Way*. New York: A.A. Knopf, 1990.

Mishra, Rammurti S., M.D. *Fundamentals of Yoga*. New York: Harmony Books, 1987.

Monro, Robin, R. Nagaranthna, and H.R. Nagendra. *Yoga for Common Ailments*. New York: Fireside, 1990.

Moyers, Bill. *Healing and the Mind*. New York: Doubleday, 1993.

O'Brien, Paddy. *Yoga for Women: Complete Mind and Body Fitness*. London: Thorsons, 1994.

Prabhupada, A.C. and Swami Bhaktivedanta. *Bhagavad-Gita As It Is*. Los Angeles: Bhaktivedanta Book Trust, 1968.

Rama, Swami. *Living With the Himalayan Masters*. Honesdale, Pennsylvania: The Himalayan Institute Press, 1999.

——. *Path of Fire and Light*. Honesdale, Pennsylvania: The Himalayan Institute Press, 1996.

Ramayana (numerous translations available).

Ravindra, Ravi. *Christ the Yogi*. Rochester, Vermont: Inner Traditions, 1998.

Rieker, Hans-Ulrich. *The Yoga of Light: Hatha Yoga Pradipika*. Middletown, California: The Dawn House Press, 1971.

Rig-Veda (multiple translations available)

Rush, Anne Kent. *The Modern Book of Yoga*. New York: Dell Publishing, 1996.

Scaravelli, Vanda. *Awakening the Spine*. New York: Harper Collins Publishers, 1991.

Schatz, Mary Pullig, M.D. *Back Care Basics*. Berkeley, California: Rodnell Press, 1992.

Schiffmann, Erich. *Yoga: The Spirit and Practice of Moving Into Stillness*. New York: Pocket Books, 1996.

Sivananda Yoga Vedanta Center. *Learn Yoga in a Weekend*. New York: Alfred A. Knopf, 1995.

——. *The Sivananda Companion to Yoga*. New York: Simon & Schuster, 1983.

——. *Yoga Mind Body*. New York: Dorling Kindersley, 1996.

Stewart, Mary and Kathy Phillips. *Yoga for Children*. London: Webster's International Publishers, 1992.

Takoma, Geo and Eve Adamson. *The Complete Idiot's Guide to Power Yoga*. Indianapolis, Indiana: Alpha Books, 1999.

Tigunait, Pandit Rajmani. *Inner Quest: The Path of Spiritual Unfoldment.* Honesdale, Pennsylvania: Yoga International Books, 1995.

Upanishads (multiple translations available)

Vishnudevananda, Swami. *The Complete Illustrated Book of Yoga.* New York: Bell Publishers, 1960.

Yogananda, Paramahansa. *Autobiography of a Yogi.* Los Angeles: Self-Realization Fellowship, 1946.

——. *Journey to Self-Realization: Discovering the Gifts of the Soul.* Los Angeles: Self Realization Fellowship, 1997.

Yogi Bhajan, Ph.D. *Kundalini Yoga, The Flow of Eternal Power.* Los Angeles: Time Capsule Books, 1996.

Yukteswar, Swami Sri. *The Holy Science.* Los Angeles: Self-Realization Fellowship, 1949.

Index

More Quality Books and Tapes
by Joan Budilovsky

Special Offer for Readers of *The Complete Idiot's Guide to Yoga, Second Edition*

Beach Blanket Yoga $7.50

Yoga fun in the sun! Live audio recording along the beautiful Chicago shoreline. Side A: Joan guides you through 30 minutes of yoga postures. Side B: Windy City waves to meditate by.

Additional Tapes and Books

Yoga Audios

Beginning Yoga with Joan $10.00

An hour of relaxing yet invigorating postures and breathwork.

Breathworks! $10.00

Thirty minutes of yoga deep-breathing exercises.

Sun-Salutations! with Joan $10.00

A dynamic series of yoga postures with meditation exercises.

Total Relaxation with Shavasana $10.00

Shavasana + Meditation = BLISS.

Yoga Books

The Little Yogi Water Book $8.00

Splish, splash, and learn water yoga with Joan.

The Little Yogi Energy Book $8.00

Energize yourself with these terrific chakra postures.

Yoga for a New Day $10.00

Yoga philosophy plus postures.

Fat-Free Yoga $8.00

Basic yoga postures and principles.

Yo Joan $10.00

Thoughtful responses to your yoga questions from the popular Yoyoga! Web site.

Massage Audios

The Art of Massage Made Simple $10.50

Joan guides you in giving a full-body, one-hour massage.

Foot Massage for Body, Mind, and Sole $10.00

Relax your feet. Relax your whole body.

Massage Video

My Swedish Massage with Joan $19.50

Spirited and instructional video on many of the massage strokes featured in *The Complete Idiot's Guide to Massage*.

Come visit Joan at her Web site: www.yoyoga.com.

Order form on next page.

Yes, send me my copies of Joan's wonderful tapes and books.

Special Audio Tape Offer
❏ Beach Blanket Yoga $7.50

Yoga Audios
❏ Beginning Yoga with Joan $10.00
❏ Breathworks! $10.00
❏ Sun-Salutations! with Joan $10.00
❏ Total Relaxation with Shavasana $10.00

Yoga Books
❏ The Little Yogi Water Book $8.00
❏ The Little Yogi Energy Book $8.00
❏ Yoga for a New Day $10.00
❏ Fat-Free Yoga $8.00
❏ Yo Joan $10.00

Massage Audios
❏ The Art of Massage Made Simple $10.50
❏ Foot Massage for Body, Mind, and Sole $10.00

Massage Video
❏ My Swedish Massage with Joan $19.50

Shipping/handling charges:

Audio/Book: Add $2.50 for one or two items; add
$.50 for each additional item. $_____
Video: Add $4.50 for first video tape; add $1.00 for
each additional video tape. $_____
Outside United States: Add $5.00. $_____
                                    Subtotal $_____
Illinois residents add 6.75% sales tax. $_____
                                    TOTAL $_____

Payment to be made in U.S. funds. Prices and availability
are subject to change without notice.
❏   Check or money order enclosed.
I would like to charge to: ❏ MasterCard   ❏ Visa
Account #: _____
Expiration Date: _____
Signature: _____
Send this order form with your check, money order, or charge information to:

Yoyoga, Inc.
P.O. Box 5013
Oak Brook, IL 60522
Phone: 630-963-1906
Fax: 630-963-4001

Allow four to six weeks for delivery.
Ship to:
Name: _____
Address: _____
City, State, Zip: _____ Phone: _____

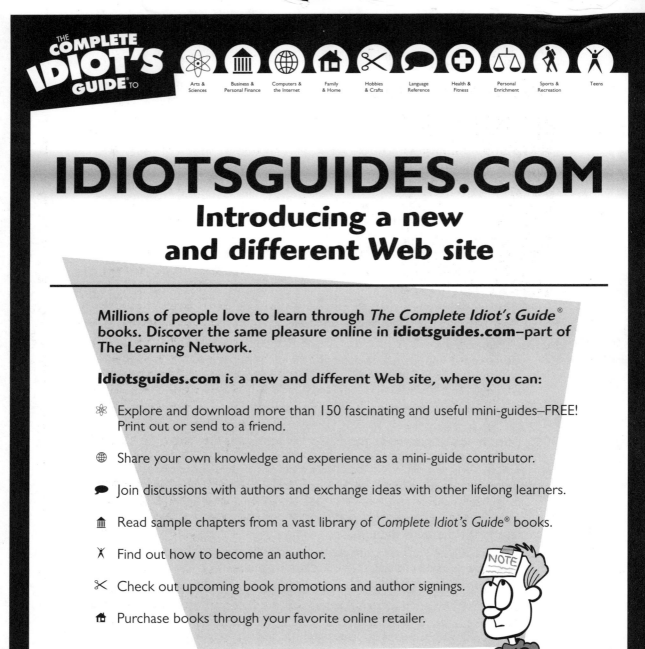